Cancer Unc

Your step-by-step guide to cancer prevention, early detection, and cancer survival.

Copyright 2012   Christopher C. Evans

ISBN: 978-1-291-23978-2

ALL RIGHTS RESERVED

First Edition.

Copyright © 2012. Christopher C. Evans
All rights reserved.

This book contains material protected under International and Federal Copyright laws and Treaties. Any unauthorised reprint or use of this material is prohibited.

Unauthorised duplication or distribution of this material in any form is strictly prohibited. Violators will be prosecuted to the fullest extent of the law. No part of this publication may be reproduced, stored in a retrieval system or transmitted in any form or by any means, electronic, mechanical, photocopying, recording or otherwise, without prior written permission from the author/publisher.

The author, publisher, and distributor of this product assume no responsibility for the use or misuse of this product, or for any physical or mental injury, damage and/or financial loss sustained to persons or property as a result of using this system. The liability, negligence, use, misuse or abuse of the operation of any methods, strategies, instructions or ideas contained in the material herein is the sole responsibility of the reader.

The material contained in this publication is provided for information purposes only. It does not diagnose nor treat any condition, nor replace sound medical advice from your doctor. (However, I would recommend that you always get a second opinion!).

Table of Contents

Foreword 9
Introduction 13
Prevention Versus Survival 22
The Basics 23
Food sources for optimal health and well-being 29
A-Z of Super Foods 30
   Açai Berries 30
   Almonds 31
   Amaranth (Amaranthus) 33
   Apples 35
   Apricots 37
   Asparagus 39
   Avocados 40
   Bananas 42
   Barley 43
   Beans 44
   Beetroot, or beets 45
   Berries 47
   Blackberries 47
   Blueberries 48
   Brazil Nuts 49
   Broccoli 50
   Cabbage 52
   Carrots 54
   Cauliflower 55
   Celery 56
   Cheese 57
   Cherries 59
   Chili Peppers 60
   Chocolate 62
   Citrus fruit 63
   Coconut oil. 64
   Cranberries 66
   Cruciferous vegetables 67
   Dark green leafy vegetables 68
   Eggs (Free Range and preferably organic). 69

- Fennel ... 71
- Figs ... 72
- Fish ... 73
- Flaxseed or Linseed ... 75
- Garlic ... 77
- Ginger Root ... 79
- Goji Berries ... 80
- Grapefruit ... 81
- Grapes and grape juice ... 83
- Green Tea ... 84
- Hazelnuts ... 86
- Honey ... 87
- Jalapeños ... 90
- Kale ... 90
- Kidney Beans ... 91
- Kiwifruit ... 92
- Lemons ... 93
- Liquorice / Licorice ... 95
- Mangoes ... 96
- Mint ... 97
- Mushrooms ... 98
- Nuts and seeds ... 100
- Olive oil ... 100
- Onions ... 102
- Oranges ... 103
- Papayas ... 104
- Parsley ... 105
- Persimmons ... 106
- Pistachio Nuts ... 107
- Pomegranates ... 108
- Potatoes ... 109
- Probiotics and Prebiotics ... 109
- Prunes ... 111
- Pumpkin and pumpkin seeds ... 112
- Raspberries ... 113
- Red grapes, red wine and grape juice ... 115
- Rice (Brown Rice) ... 116
- Rosemary ... 117
- Rye ... 119
- Seaweed ... 120
- Sesame seeds ... 123

Soy 124
Spinach 127
Strawberries.. 129
Sunflower seeds 130
Sweet Potatoes 131
Tomatoes 132
Turmeric 134
Walnuts.. 136
Water.. 137
Watercress 138
Whey... 139
Whole Grains 142

Foods to Avoid 144
Alcohol 144
Artificial sweeteners 145
Caffeine / Coffee.. 153
Processed meats 154
Dairy products... 156
Genetically Modified Foods (GMOs) 159
Hydrogenated fats and trans fats 166
Acrylamide.. 167
Monosodium glutamate.. 169
Preservatives, including phosphates 172
Pickled foods 174
Refined sugar and sugar alcohols.. 174
Very hot tea.. 180
Wheat 181
Junk food 185

Anticancer Activities 187
Enjoy Exercise.. 187
Seek out moderate sun exposure... 189
Get plenty of sleep... 190
Colonic massage... 191
(Men) Sit down to use the toilet.. 193
Dry skin brushing... 194
Far-Infrared sauna.. 198
Meditation 199
Socialising... 201

Environmental Factors to Avoid 202
Smoking (or use of tobacco in any form) 202

5

Wearing a bra?..203
Excessive sun exposure or excessive suntan lotion exposure?......206
Radon gas...207
Radiation and magnetic fields 208
   Mobile Telephones..*208*
   Power Lines..*209*
   CT scans, x-rays and mammograms *211*
Known conditions that contribute to cancer risk 213
Diesel/petrol and exhaust fumes..214
Carcinogens..215
Aluminium-based antiperspirants and deodorants (US spelling - Aluminum) 216
Allergens / food intolerances 218
Illegal Drugs..223
Dental toxicity...225
Heavy metals 229
Parasites..232
Sunbeds and Fake Tan..236
Pesticides and herbicides..238
Bisphenol A in plastics 240
Toxins we cannot avoid 243

Cancer Survival Psychology 245
Is survival a state of mind?..245
Is laughter the best medicine? 245
Support and relationships 248
Socialising...249
The placebo effect 251
Emotional stress and depression..254
Unresolved emotional issues and suppressed emotions.................256
Look for the good in cancer..258

Early Detection 259
Look for any changes in your health 259
Self-examinations:..260
   Testicular self-examination:...*260*
   Breast self-examination: *261*
   Skin self-examination: *264*
   Blood tests to detect or monitor cancer.......................................*265*
   Medical imaging..*266*
   Other diagnostic procedures *267*

Cancer Information 273

Cancer Research 274

Cancer Treatment 279

"Alternative" Medicine 290
What do we know about cancer?.................................. 291
Dr Krebs and Vitamin B17... 293
Dr Burzynski and Antineoplastons 296
Dr Issels and Issels Integrative Oncology................... 297
Dr Coley and Coley's Vaccine.. 299
Dr Johanna Budwig - The Budwig Diet....................... 302
Dr Gerson and Gerson Therapy 306
Dr Andrew Ivy and Krebiozen 312
Dr Burton's IAT - Immuno-Augmentative Therapy ... 316
Dr. Royal R. Rife - every disease has a frequency...... 320
Dr. William Koch and Glyoxylide 323
Ozone therapy and Oxygen Therapy........................... 329
Dietary and intravenous vitamin C or ascorbic acid... 330
Hyperthermia.. 337
Proteolytic enzymes... 338
Pancreatic enzymes... 338
Alkaline Water.. 339
Alkaline Forming Foods.. 341
Insulin Potentiation... 345
Metronomic Treatment... 345
Rick Simpson and hemp oil 347
Further reading.. 350

Conclusion 351

The Lazy Guide To Cancer Prevention 354
Food sources you should eat daily................................ 354
Food sources you should eat less of, or avoid.............. 356
Habits and environmental factors you should seek more of......... 357
Habits and environmental factors you should seek to avoid........ 358
Using your psychology to give you the edge................ 358

The Dedicated Guide To Cancer Prevention 360
Food sources you should eat daily................................ 360
Food sources you should eat less of, or avoid.............. 363
Habits and environmental factors you should seek more of......... 364
Habits and environmental factors you should seek to avoid........ 365
Using your psychology to give you the edge................ 366

The Survivors Guide To Cancer Prevention and Survival....... 367
Food sources you should eat daily 367
Food sources you should eat less of, or avoid. 370
Habits and environmental factors you should seek more of. 371
Habits and environmental factors you should seek to avoid..........372
Using your psychology to give you the edge..............................373
Alternative Therapy Checklist 374

Foreword

This book came about through my 17 years of experience in medical diagnostics and an intense fascination with nutrition and all things biological.

To put my passion in perspective, when I was just 15 years old, I was already taking evening classes in A level biology for the sheer love of the subject... and my leisure reading included medical text books such as Grey's Anatomy!

So when writing this book, I wanted to share that passion, by explaining the little things that people can easily do to make a big difference in their cancer risk. Simple daily strategies that could save lives.

I supposed that if the strategies I recommended were difficult, then many people simply wouldn't implement them. So I set out to make this as painless as possible!

I must say that until a week ago, writing this book was primarily an intellectual experience for me. I had seen many other authors citing very emotional triggers for their research, such as family members being diagnosed with cancer, (or bereavements), but in my case it was born from a love of science and the drive to help people...

...But less than a week before my book launch, my wife was told by her Doctor that she had cancer. A bombshell right out of the blue.

I have had well over a decade of wanting to put this book together, without my acting upon that impulse. But over the last three months I felt increasingly driven to complete it. I worked all hours, researching and dictating, with a feverish passion to get this book finished. Often putting in 20 hour days and jeopardising my own health in order to get it completed - all without even the slightest knowledge that my wife was ill.

Is it pure coincidence that my wife's cancer diagnosis came now? Was it fate? Or was I being driven by a higher power to be as well informed as possible, so I could help her? I simply don't know.

But the fact remains that I could have written my book at ANY time in the last 10 years.

Do you believe in serendipity? The timing seemed very strange to me, so I did some calculations on the probability of these two independent events happening together.

If you take it that one of these events was fixed in time, i.e. predetermined, then over a 10 year period, the chance of writing my book within the same 3 month window as my wife's cancer diagnosis is just a 2.5% probability or a 1 in 40 chance. (Because there are 40 x 3 month blocks of time within a 10 year period, and it could have happened in any one of them).

But on the same basis, the probability of her diagnosis being within just 1 week of my publishing date is just a miniscule 0.19% probability, not even a fifth of 1 percent. Just 1 in 520 chance. (1 week out of 520 possible weeks).

If you take it that either event might, or might not, have happened at any time in the last 10 years, then the chance of them BOTH happening within the exact same week is 1 in 270,400!

I don't know what to make of that myself, because coincidences do happen. But I am an optimistic person by nature, so if I were to assign it meaning, it would have a very positive connotation.

Either way, in the blink of an eye, my intellectual and creative experience has been brutally converted into an emotional one. It is only upon being so intimately involved with cancer that you begin to remotely understand what other people are going through every single day.

With this in mind, if you are reading this book for prevention, then spare a moment to consider the devastating impact that a diagnosis can have on yourself and your family, and use this to motivate yourself towards making a solid effort at prevention.

If you have already been diagnosed, or if one of your loved ones has, then please accept my absolute, sincere and heart-felt condolences, and accept my urge for you to put this information into daily practice, just as we have.

Whilst this information is scientifically sound and supported by numerous peer-reviewed scientific studies, we too feel the trepidation of having to put it all into practice with no guarantee of success.

But we are embracing it fully, and taking every step we can to support my wife's body's natural ability to fight the cancer. We will combine the best parts of conventional medicine with complementary medicine and good nutrition.

Finally, I would like to thank all of the contributors to this book, along with my office staff, who have been very patient and held the fort whilst I was engrossed in completing this task. I would specifically like to thank Richard Davies for his proofreading skills, and Sarah Hall for proofreading and providing the images and cover artwork.

Most of all, I would like to thank my wife, Lisa, for giving me the time-freedom to write the book, and for sharing the experience we are both facing. I have never known someone so stoic and cheerful in the face of adversity. She is a real inspiration to me.

I fully intend to embrace every moment, whether it is spending precious time together, or learning new life lessons.

Regardless of our lot in life, I think it is fundamental that we learn to embrace the lessons life has to offer, that we retain a sense of gratitude, that we continue to grow, and that we love one another.

I hope this book gives you a sense of hope and helps you to focus on the precious gift of LIFE.

Introduction

This book is about your survival. On that basis, it deliberately pulls no punches. We live in an environment where cancer levels are increasing daily, despite the efforts of mainstream medicine.

The base reality is that cancer is largely preventable and that the exact same preventative steps can also be used to significantly increase the chance of your survival if you are diagnosed.

The US alone has spent in excess of $400 billion in cancer research, with literally thousands of studies concluded worldwide, and yet our mainstream treatment methods have barely changed to reflect the new data. In fact, data shows that many mainstream approaches kill as many people as they save.

In this book, you will learn the key facts that the studies have highlighted - the simple actions you can take, and changes you can make, to decrease your risk of cancer many times over, or else to greatly increase your chances of survival if you have already been diagnosed.

In order to make the best use of this book, you will need to adjust your mindset to take into account the following:

1. **The fields of cancer research and treatment are hugely political** and support an industry with an annual turnover exceeding three quarters of a TRILLION dollars worldwide. Idealists would like to see a cure for cancer, but the cure would slash the bottom line of one of the planet's largest industries. This is bound to influence the choices that the industry makes and their attitude towards solutions that cannot easily be monetised.
2. **Your Doctor does not know everything.** After Medical school, your Doctor stays abreast of the latest research via medical journals which are largely funded by the pharmaceutical industry. These journals are biased in

favour of mainstream medicine because it promotes the pharmaceutical products that pay for the Journal's existence. Of course your doctor plays a vital role, but you must educate yourself and question their recommendations.
3. **Less than 2% of cancer research is devoted to prevention** even though it is widely acknowledged that 85% of cancer is preventable.
4. **Preventing cancer and helping your body to fight it (if you have been diagnosed), are largely the same process.**

The first step is understanding that you cannot focus purely on cancer without first addressing the wider perspective of your general health.

Therefore, the information presented within this book is not only aimed at improving your odds of survival where cancer is concerned, but it also addresses your energy levels, general health and well-being and can have an impact upon many other conditions such as heart disease, diabetes, obesity, depression and more.

I would hope that you would attack this material with veracity, as it carries within it the statistical probability of adding years to your life-span. Years to be spent with loved ones, enjoying retirement, and fulfilling your potential.

However, I am a realist. Life gets in the way and some of the studies presented in the book highlight action steps requiring more effort than others.

On that basis, whilst I provide what I believe to be the complete picture, at the conclusion of this book I have created several cheat sheets containing the actions you need to take. These have been divided into three subcategories, to suit three levels of dedication to this process:

1. The Lazy Guide, (the easiest and yet most effective strategies).

2. The Dedicated Guide, (additional strategies to give you the edge, whilst still being reasonably practical).

3. The Survivor's Guide, (every single strategy which holds credibility that can be used synergistically to maximise your chance of survival. This is for those who will do whatever it takes to minimise their risk of cancer or to fight back beyond diagnosis).

I appreciate that there is a lot of information already available on the subject, but unfortunately, some of it is conflicting, some of it is hard to substantiate with empirical evidence and a significant proportion of it has been generated whilst simultaneously furthering the vested interests of the drug companies who make billions from this condition.

It has taken considerable research to draw out the common threads associated with survival and longevity, but this book is the culmination of that research process. I have done the work so that you don't have to, and make it accessible in one place for your easy consumption.

As time goes on, and as new study data becomes available, I shall endeavour to keep this work current and up to date, but in the interim please take action. Not a lethargic, half-hearted "I'm too busy" action, but vigorous, dedicated and daily action to hold onto the most precious gifts you have - HEALTH and TIME.

In fact, get **angry**. Emotion drives us to action and a brief shot of anger yields to **determination**. Refuse to settle for ill-health, reduced life-span, lower levels of energy and the inability to participate in LIFE. Cancer is a legacy that has been handed down to people through society-driven changes in the environment, diet, lifestyle choices, blinkered medicine and more - but you do not have to accept it. Just say NO! - and mean it!

Based upon the data I will present, you will see that cancer, for the most part, is a consequence of what your body has been exposed to through your diet and the environment - less than 10% of cancer is related to your genetic predisposition. All you need is the right information, the right research and the right plan of action to change the options available to you.

Nobody can guarantee a cure, and nobody can guarantee prevention. However, statistically, the vast majority of cases could be prevented and there are known factors that hinder the development and growth of cancer when you have it. This is where both you and I will focus our energy.

It is time to get serious. It is time to SURVIVE.

Cancer in the 21st-Century

Many people do not realise it, but cancer is a modern disease of our own making. The fields of Egyptology, Archaeology and the resulting research have shown us that out of literally hundreds, (if not thousands) of mummified bodies studied, (many of which using modern imaging equipment) only a single mummy with cancer has ever been discovered. The causes of death have been well documented, and yet no cancer. In ancient Greek and Roman literature, cancer was virtually unheard of.

Research carried out at Manchester's KNH Centre for Biomedical Egyptology, and published in Nature Reviews Cancer was reported as follows:

"Cancer is a modern, man-made disease caused by environmental factors such as pollution and diet, a study review by University of Manchester scientists has strongly suggested.

Their study of remains and literature from ancient Egypt and Greece and earlier periods – includes the first histological diagnosis of cancer in an Egyptian mummy.

Finding only one case of the disease in the investigation of hundreds of Egyptian mummies, with few references to cancer in literary evidence, proves that cancer was extremely rare in antiquity. The disease rate has risen massively since the Industrial Revolution, in particular childhood cancer – proving that the rise is not simply due to people living longer.

Professor Rosalie David, at the Faculty of Life Sciences, said: "In industrialised societies, cancer is second only to cardiovascular disease as a cause of death. But in ancient times, it was extremely rare. There is nothing in the natural environment that can cause [the current level of] cancer. So it has to be a man-made disease, down to pollution and changes to our diet and lifestyle."

She added: "The important thing about our study is that it gives a historical perspective to this disease. We can make very clear statements on the cancer rates in societies because we have a full overview. We have looked at millennia, not one hundred years, and have masses of data."

The data includes the first ever histological diagnosis of cancer in an Egyptian mummy by Professor Michael Zimmerman, a visiting Professor at the KNH Centre, who is based at the Villanova University in the US. He diagnosed rectal cancer in an unnamed mummy, an 'ordinary' person who had lived in the Dakhleh Oasis during the Ptolemaic period (200-400 CE).

Professor Zimmerman said: "In an ancient society lacking surgical intervention, evidence of cancer should remain in all cases. The virtual absence of malignancies in mummies must be interpreted as indicating their rarity in antiquity, indicating that cancer causing factors are limited to societies affected by modern industrialization".

The team studied both mummified remains and literary evidence for ancient Egypt but only literary evidence for ancient Greece as there are no remains for this period, as well as medical studies of human and animal remains from earlier periods, going back to the age of the dinosaurs.

It has been suggested that the short life span of individuals in antiquity precluded the development of cancer. Although this statistical construct is true, individuals in ancient Egypt and Greece did live long enough to develop such diseases as atherosclerosis, Paget's disease of bone, and osteoporosis, and, in modern populations, bone tumours primarily affect the young." - Manchester University.

You can see evidence of the gradual increase in cancer rates across all cancers. For example, in 1940, approximately 1 in 20 women in the US would be diagnosed with breast cancer within their lifetimes, but more recently, it has been estimated as being approximately 1 in 8.

Currently, 1 in 3 people in the US will get cancer in their lifetimes and in the next 15 to 20 years it is predicted that this will increase to 1 in 2. The numbers have been drastically rising since the Industrial Revolution - which corresponds to the dramatic increase in pollution, the increase in population size and the resultant requirement for mass-produced, cheap sources of food (particularly in the last 50 to 60 years). Combine this with the 21st-century sedentary lifestyle and the massive commercialisation of the agricultural industry and you soon have a strong case that, as a society, we are fostering an environment conducive to the development of ill-health and cancer.

The Western world is now spending more money on healthcare than ever before, and yet our success rates have either remained the same since the beginning, or even decreased. I fully appreciate the dedication (and genuine drive to help patients) of your average medical practitioner, but the system is broken and perspective has been lost.

In fact, according to data from a range of peer-reviewed medical journals, and research by Gary Null PhD, Carolyn Dean MD ND, Martin Feldman MD, Debora Rasio MD and Dorothy Smith PhD, it is apparent that by 2001, the American health care system was the number one cause of death in America!

So much for Florence Nightingale's maxim of "first do no harm." That year, the US annual death rate from heart disease was 699,697 and the annual death rate from cancer was 553,251. But deaths brought about directly by the US healthcare system came to 783,936 that same year. (Adverse Drug Reactions 106,000, Medical error 98,000, Bedsores 115,000, Hospital infections 88,000, Malnutrition 108,800, Outpatients 199,000, Unnecessary Procedures 37,136, Surgery-Related 32,000).

So as heroic as individual doctors can be, the underlying system of Western medicine is failing in numerous areas.

Thomas Edison once said:

"The doctor of the future will no longer treat the human frame with drugs, but rather will cure and prevent disease with nutrition."

All those years ago, Edison, with his extraordinary ability to innovate and see directly to the heart of the problem, could see the direction that modern medicine needed to follow.

And sure enough, contemporary medical research across countless clinical studies, has shown that modifications to your diet can drastically reduce the chances of you getting cancer, whilst simultaneously increasing your likelihood of survival if you have already been diagnosed.

Perhaps this is simple logic: give your body the raw building blocks it needs to maintain a healthy immune system, endocrine (hormonal) system, and normal body weight, whilst avoiding the cancer-causing agents in our environment. Add regular exercise (which helps your lymphatic system to move its fluids around your body, boosting your immune system) and you have eliminated well over 85% of the causes of cancer.

Unfortunately, as you will see in later chapters, the pharmaceutical industry, the food industry, the chemical industry, (to name but a few), have extraordinary vested interests in promoting their products even at the expense of the consumer and the wider public interest, and this makes the avoidance of carcinogenic substances almost, (but not entirely), impossible.

At risk of promoting conspiracy theories, I'll explain the background of some of these vested interests, along with the public consequences. Unfortunately, much of the information I will present goes well beyond theory.

I am reminded of a quote by George Orwell:

"During times of universal deceit, telling the truth becomes a revolutionary act."

On this basis, and without further ado, I propose to lay out the raw data, for your evaluation, followed by the precise action steps you need to take, in the form of step-by-step cheat sheets.

How to consume this material

For those of you who are too impatient to evaluate the background evidence, I have created three cheat sheets. The lazy guide, the dedicated guide and the survivor's guide. Feel free to cut to the chase to see exactly what you should be doing in order to stay healthy, (or to improve your health). However, I would caution that unless you understand the background reasoning for these items, and unless you have experienced the immersion of reading through the entire book, you may perhaps be less inclined to stick rigidly to the plan.

So please take the time to consume this material in the order it was written so that you can build a foundation, not only in terms of logical scientific data, but also within your emotional journey of change. Because change is absolutely necessary. I would not suggest that the changes are not beneficial, nor that they cannot be enjoyed, but it is human nature to get stuck in a rut and prefer things exactly how you like them. This is not always in your best interests.

With such a radical increase in the risk factors associated with cancer, you need an equally radical change in your habits, diet, lifestyle and understanding of health (and psychology).

"Let food be thy medicine and medicine be thy food" - Hippocrates

Prevention Versus Survival

Whilst I have provided sections specifically on cancer treatment and alternative medicine, I firmly believe that the same identical steps taken for prevention, have a massive impact on survival rates.

Therefore whether you are a currently diagnosed cancer patient, somebody in remission, or simply somebody who is proactively making improvements on their health, the same information is valid and should be put into practice.

Furthermore, if you have already been diagnosed, or are in remission, I would strongly advocate that you get fanatical about your health. Do your best to follow my "Survivors guide", to give your body, mind and spirit every opportunity to thrive and survive.

"Health is like money, we never have a true idea of its value until we lose it." - Josh Billings

By the same token, if you have a strong family history of cancer, then you too should certainly attempt to follow my "Dedicated guide", if not the more in-depth "Survivors guide". A family history of cancer isn't always about genetics, because you are probably eating out of the same refrigerator, adopting the same eating habits and exercise patterns. If you change those factors, you are likely to change the outcome.

Some of the study data I present even shows dramatic reduction in levels of cancer risk in those with genetic predisposition. It is all down to setting yourself up for success by doing and eating the right things.

"Time and health are two precious assets that we don't recognize and appreciate until they have been depleted." - Denis Waitley.

The Basics

I do not wish to assume that as a reader, you have any prior knowledge of nutritional science. At best, most individuals have been exposed to a smattering of educational marketing from television commercials, or basic information from their science classes at school or college. On that basis, I should provide you with the fundamentals:

In order to survive, we require certain raw materials to be consumed in the form of food. These raw materials give us energy, the fundamental building blocks upon which our body is built, and the necessary chemicals to sustain our metabolic processes. At the most basic level, the foods we consume are split into three main macronutrients:

Carbohydrates - typically associated with easily utilisable energy in the form of sugars or starches. I am sure you will have heard of complex carbohydrates, which are supposed to release energy more slowly than say, raw sugar, because they take your body longer to break them down. Examples of foods high in carbohydrates include: sugar, rice, flour, potato, pasta, etc.

Fats - lipid-based stores of energy, such as oils and hard fats. I am sure you have heard of saturated and unsaturated fats. Fats are very calorie dense. i.e a small amount of fat contains a lot of calories - 1g of fat contains 9 calories of energy, whereas 1g of carbohydrates only contains 4 calories of energy. Most importantly, whilst modern marketing has demonised fats (because they contain higher calorific values) and promoted everything "low-fat" or "non-fat", the right kinds of fats are **very** important to your body and should not be ignored. Many of the vitamins and minerals you need are fat-soluble, or are transported into the body using fat. Examples of fats include: lard, vegetable oil, olive oil, and foods high in fat such as cream or cheese.

Protein - proteins are comprised of sub-units called amino acids. Protein provides the fundamental building blocks of material that most of your tissues are made from. Protein isn't just present in muscle - it is present in your ligaments, tendons, skin, organs, hair and pretty much every other tissue. You also have proteins in your bodily fluids acting as enzymes within your body. Enzymes enable chemical reactions to take place, which are necessary for life and the proper functioning of every cell in your body. Examples of sources of protein include: meat, fish, poultry, nuts, eggs, whey, milk, etc.

In terms of the micronutrients, you often hear of vitamins and minerals (which we will go in to), but you do not hear much about phytochemicals, plant sterols, enzymes, etc.

This lack of general understanding is a real problem, because people assume that eating their processed, irradiated, freeze-dried, pasteurised, preserved convenience foods will cut it. Often they just provide hollow calories with almost no nutritional value.

Let me put it to you this way. In the food industry, a lot of effort goes towards finding better ways of preserving produce. This allows food to fare better when being transported, it allows a greater shelf life for convenience, and minimises waste for the stores.

However, the natural process of decomposition within food is brought about by the enzymes within it. The same enzymes that enable you to break down and digest the food in an efficient manner when it enters your body. Without those enzymes your body has to work a lot harder to generate its own, and may not entirely break the food down.

When foods have been irradiated, packed with preservatives, heat-treated and more, the processing disables these naturally occurring and vital enzymes. This makes the food last longer, however it also largely accounts for why the average 50-year-old American has upwards of 10 lbs of toxic, compacted fecal matter lining their digestive tract. Scary but true. A low-fiber and meat-rich diet is a significant contributor, but increasing your consumption of enzyme-rich foods will certainly help to reduce that toxic burden over time.

Bowel cancer levels are currently at an all-time high, and even those without that condition are taxing their immune systems and allowing their blood to carry higher levels of toxins than they need to.

It is no wonder that we have problems when you look at the western diet. In 2009, the American Cancer Association found that only 23.8% of American adults consume 5 or more portions of fruit or vegetables each day. That is less than one quarter of the population!

So, is all processed food bad? Well, even when long-life foods have been fortified with certain vitamins and minerals (or essential fatty acids) by the manufacturers (often for marketing purposes), your body cannot always use them fully - because they do not have the natural balance of nutrients your body needs.

For example, various foods have been fortified with additional omega-3 essential fatty acids. Manufacturers will tell you that this is great for brain development, attention span and learning in children, (and many foods are now depleted of this type of fat), but what the manufacturers do not tell you is that your child also needs omega-6 essential fatty acids in their diet to make use of omega-3! Ideally, you want equal parts of Omega-3 and Omega-6 in your diet.

Such gimics are perhaps misleading to the consumer, but are allowed because they comply with labeling requirements and advertising standards.

By the same token, it also isn't very well-publicised that in battery hen eggs (where the caged hen is fed nothing but commercial hen feed) the omega-3 to omega-6 ratio is around 1 to 20. However, the ratio of an egg from an organic free range hen (which is allowed to eat natural produce) is around 20 to 20. This means that your body can utilise up to 20 times more of the omega-3 and omega-6 essential fatty acids. In isolation, you would have to eat almost 20 mass produced battery hen eggs to get the same nutritional benefits!

The average Western diet has a ratio of around 15 parts of omega-6 to 1 part omega-3. According to The Center for Genetics, Nutrition and Health, Washington, DC 20009, USA, "such a high ratio has been shown to increase the likelihood of "many diseases, including cardiovascular disease, cancer, and inflammatory and autoimmune diseases, whereas increased levels of omega-3 (a low omega-6/omega-3 ratio) exert suppressive effects.

In the secondary prevention of cardiovascular disease, a ratio of 4/1 was associated with a 70% decrease in total mortality. A ratio of 2.5/1 reduced rectal cell proliferation in patients with colorectal cancer"... "The lower omega-6/omega-3 ratio in women with breast cancer was associated with decreased risk. A ratio of 2-3/1 suppressed inflammation in patients with rheumatoid arthritis, and a ratio of 5/1 had a beneficial effect on patients with asthma."

These are very interesting results, and yet how many cancer patients have been told to increase their omega-3 intake by their doctors? This is the same with so many other nutrients, despite solid study data backing their potential for reducing the risk of cancer.

Nutrition is the elephant in the room that the cancer research and medical communities are studiously ignoring. You cannot afford to do the same.

"The best doctor gives the least medicines." - Benjamin Franklin

In the case of processed food, the enzymes that your body would use to digest the food (to make use of all of the goodness it contains) can be virtually absent. This means that the burden to produce them rests entirely on your body - which is already overtaxed from dealing with the buildup of waste you have been accumulating, probably over the last several decades.

Such processed food is almost biochemically dead. So what is the solution? The closer your food is to fresh and raw, the more non-synthesizable phytonutrients and enzymes are still within it.

To put it in perspective your body utilises over 5000 different enzymes and these do not come out of a vitamin pill or microwaveable ready meal. Many of these live plant-based compounds are simply not present in anything but fresh raw foods.

Even a vitamin tablet is of limited value if the vitamins within it are not provided in the most bioavailable format, and if you do not have reserves of the necessary enzymes to use them, nor the right fats in your diet to help transport them across the gut into your bloodstream. Nutrients consumed in the wrong quantities or without the correct balance of other supporting nutrients and enzymes are simply adding to the burden of waste your body needs to remove. So we need to get smart about what we put into our bodies.

A significant proportion of the current obesity crisis is the fact that nutritionally, many people are effectively starving to death. There is no problem with an abundance of fast-food calories, but the nutritional value of the foods that the average person consumes are so poor that their bodies are in a constant state of craving.

Even with the best will in the world, a solid basis of scientific knowledge and a good budget, it can still be difficult to consume sufficient nutrition because the intensive farming methods used over the last 50 to 60 years have depleted the nutrients from the topsoil of farmland.

So this book is designed to help you optimise what you eat. Don't worry, you have the answers within these pages, but as much as I would like you to obtain your nutrition from fresh produce, it may not be entirely possible to reach optimum levels without supplementation.

Let me give you a good example. Many people remember Popeye the sailor, a popular cartoon character from 1929 onwards. Whenever anything went horribly wrong, and Popeye was required to come to the rescue, he would pop open a can of spinach, swallow it down and develop super strength in order to save the day.

Back in the 1940s, a can of spinach contained 158mg of iron. By 1965, the same can of spinach only contained 27mg of iron. Fast forward to the present day, and the same can of spinach may contain as little as 2mg of iron, meaning that Popeye would have to consume a whopping 79 cans of spinach before he could come to the rescue!

I don't know about you, but I would pretty well give up on him getting there in time!

So, what is the solution? By consuming foods that are naturally super-rich in vitamins, minerals, essential fatty acids and the natural active plant compounds and enzymes, we can give ourselves a good basis for nutrition. This can be further improved by consuming organic produce, which has not had the same commercial stripping of nutrition from the land, nor the harmful pesticides and herbicides that can contaminate the food. This can further be boosted with low-cost supplementation of vitamins, minerals, essential fatty acids, probiotics and enzymes.

With that in mind, the following sections include:

- Food sources you should eat more of (The A-Z of super foods).

- Food sources you should eat less of, or avoid.

- Habits and environmental factors you should seek more of.

- Habits and environmental factors you should seek to avoid.

- Using your psychology to give you the edge.

Food sources for optimal health and well-being

"Today, more than 95% of all chronic disease is caused by food choice, toxic food ingredients, nutritional deficiencies and lack of physical exercise." - Mike Adams

The following foods should be consumed as your first choice. These foods may not always be convenient, but the advantage is that most of them can be eaten raw or require minimal preparation.

As a rule of thumb, as much as 80% of your diet should be consumed as close to raw as possible. This preserves the delicate enzymes and active compounds present within the food.

If you do eat cooked food, then at least supplement the meal with digestive enzyme capsules to take the burden from your body to produce enzymes, and to increase the absorption of nutrition from your food.

Visit:

http://www.CancerUncensored.com/recommended-products

"Take care of your body. It's the only place you have to live." - Jim Rohn

A-Z of Super Foods

In order to be enable easier referencing, I shall list the following foods and supplements with considerable health benefits and potential anti-cancer properties in alphabetical order:

Açai Berries

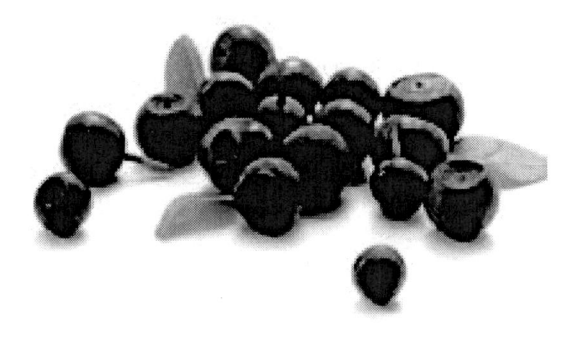

The antioxidant capacity or "ORAC" value for a 4 ounce portion of açai berries is 6576, which is greater than blueberries, strawberries and red wine combined.

Having high antioxidant value prevents damage from free radicals in your system caused by smoking, pollution and the metabolism of your food. Free radicals are atoms, molecules or ions that do not have a balanced amount of electrons, so they aggressively react with your tissues to resolve this issue. Antioxidants are able to sacrifice themselves, so that your tissues do not take damage.

Açai berries are unique to the Amazon rainforests of Brazil, where in some cities açai juice is consumed in greater quantities than milk.

Although it is a fruit, it does contain a high proportion of fat, but these are the healthy anti-inflammatory omega-9 fats that improve your cholesterol levels, boost your immune system and can improve your heart health. You can find these same fats in foods such as avocados, olive oil, sesame oil, olives and nuts (almonds, peanuts, pecans, pistachios, hazelnuts, cashews and macadamia).

In addition to the high levels of anthocyanins (which act as antioxidants and provide a number of other health benefits) açai also contain phytosterols that help to reduce cholesterol and ease the symptoms associated with benign prostatic hyperplasia (enlarged prostate).

Studies conducted by the University of Florida also showed that the powerful antioxidant compounds in açai berries reduced the rate of cell proliferation (how quickly cells multiplied), and aided apoptosis (programmed cell death) in human leukaemia cells.

Almonds

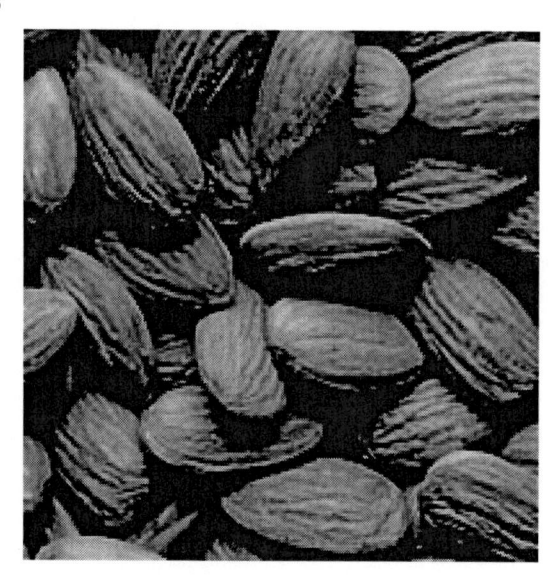

Almonds and especially almond extract contain benzaldehyde, which is shown in studies to exert an anti-cancer effect. So use almond extract to flavour drinks and find ways to include almonds in your diet.

Almonds also contain a high level of dietary fibre, which has been shown to help reduce the risk of colon/bowel cancer. They also contain calcium, magnesium, zinc, phosphorus, folic acid and vitamin E, which between them, assist your immune system, heart health and encourage the maintenance of healthy eyes, teeth and bones.

The folic acid in almonds may help reduce the risk of cervical cancers. Researchers in Finland have even linked almonds to a reduction in risk of lung cancers.

A study conducted by the University of California found that the consumption of almonds has a significant impact upon the prevention of colon cancer in rats.

In 2006, a study in the American Journal of Clinical Nutrition showed that eating almonds increased levels of cholecystokinin (CCK), which is a hormone that is associated with the satiety that you get from eating fat-rich foods. This means that after eating almonds you feel more satisfied, are less hungry and are less likely to snack.

This level of satisfaction was greater in women than men. Further studies conducted by researchers at King's College in London found that almonds may help to block the absorption of carbohydrates and improve the feeling of satiety in both men and women.

If you combine that with the 2003 study published in the International Journal of Obesity, which showed that adding three handfuls of almonds to a low-calorie diet each day significantly increased the weight loss of the participants in comparison with a low-calorie diet alone, it shows that almonds are a great addition to everybody's diet.

Almond milk is a beverage made from ground almonds, often used as a substitute for milk. Unlike animal milk, almond milk contains no cholesterol or lactose. As it does not contain any animal products, it is suitable for vegans and vegetarians who abstain from dairy products. Almond milk is much better if you blend it yourself using almonds and water. This avoids the deterioration in nutrition when the manufacturers heat treat it.

Amaranth (Amaranthus)

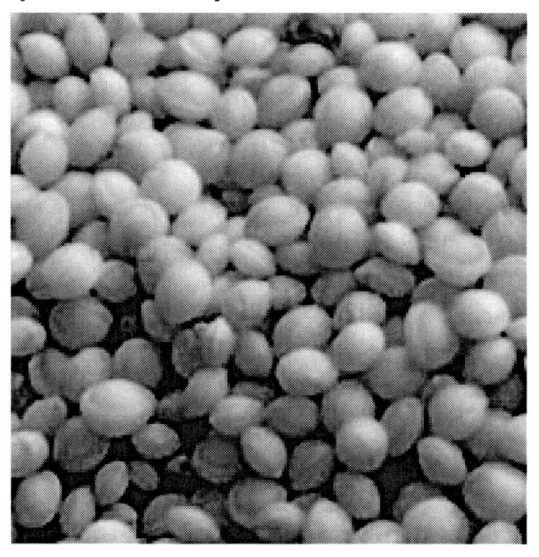

Amaranth is an ancient grain of the Aztecs, which is thought to date back as much as 8000 years ago. It was almost lost due to the conquering Spaniards burning the amaranth fields as part of their conquest.

Today, the amaranth grain is cultivated in China, Mexico, Central America and more recently in certain parts of the US including Nebraska, Illinois and Colorado.

Amaranth has the highest level of protein per serving out of all of the different grains, including an amino acid called lysine which none of the other grains have. Amaranth can be added to other plant protein sources to create whole protein, which enables humans to be vegetarian without deficiencies. It is very high in fibre, which has been shown to reduce the likelihood of bowel cancer and is a great source of iron, which enables our body to manufacture red blood cells and keep our oxygen levels high.

It also contains the cancer fighting phytochemical squalene, along with calcium, magnesium and folic acid.

In studies, the antioxidant squalene has been shown to reduce or halt the blood supply to tumours, thereby reducing their ability to grow and spread. Shark oil, only has 1% squalene content, whereas amaranth oil is 8%. Other studies also indicate that the amaranth seed can inhibit the growth of breast cancer cells.

When it comes to heart disease, amaranth is almost as effective in lowering LDL-cholesterol as oats, and in the case of diabetics, amaranth has been found to reduce the incidence of hyperglycaemia (an excess of blood sugar). In one study, that used diabetic rats, amaranth was seen to significantly decrease serum glucose, increase insulin levels and normalised elevated liver function markers.

You can use amaranth flour to add this grain to your diet, or else you can toast the seeds in a pan, which makes them pop like popcorn. This can then be added to casseroles, salads or used as a crunchy topping for soups, lasagne or even as a replacement for breadcrumbs on fish or meat.

Apples

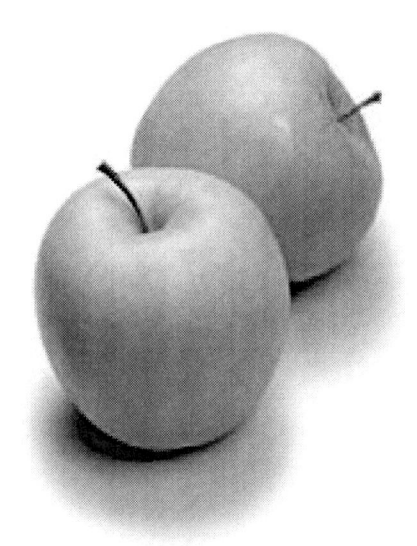

Everybody has heard the phrase "an apple a day keeps the doctor away". This is because Apples contain a wide variety of nutrients and active plant compounds.

You will probably have noticed that when you cut an apple in half, and expose it to the air, it only takes a few minutes before it starts to discolour. This is because it is rich in enzymes. Our diets do not contain enough enzymes, due to the extensive processing of food, so any enzyme-rich food sources are good news for us.

Apples also contain dietary fibre, vitamin C, phytosterols (which help reduce cholesterol), beta-carotene, a whole range of antioxidants and other vitamins and minerals.

Apples are often included in cleansing diets due to their ability to help clear toxins from the body. This is largely due to their fibre content. The fibre in apples is a water soluble fibre known as pectin, which has the ability to bind up toxins, heavy metals and the bad form of cholesterol to remove them from the body. This makes Apples not only good for your bowels, but good for your arteries.

The flavonoid quercetin, also has anti-inflammatory properties and can reduce allergic reactions.

Research at Cornell University in the US, concluded that apple consumption substantially inhibited breast tumour growth in rats. This was put down to the high concentration of phytochemicals found in apples.

The research was carried out over a 24 week period and was based on the deadliest kind of breast cancer tumour called adenocarcinoma. The greater the amount of apple extract the rats received, the better the results. The dose was matched to the human equivalent of either one, three, or six Apples daily. In the low-dose group, tumours were discovered in 57% of the rats, in the medium dose group, 50% exhibited tumours and yet in the high-dose group, only 23% of rats were found to have tumours.

Apples are a substantial source of phenolics, which are a type of phytochemical. Oranges, grapes, strawberries and plums all contain these compounds, but at a lower level.

Another interesting factor is that Apple seeds contain vitamin B17. Vitamin B17, otherwise known as Amygdalin or Laetrile is a nitriloside, which naturally occurs in a range of foods, including some berries, some beans, grasses, leaves, nuts, flax, bitter almonds, beansprouts, millet and certain fruit seeds. In fact it is found in over 1200 edible plants. It is particularly prevalent in the seeds of apples, apricots and peaches.

The subject of vitamin B17 is discussed in greater detail in the Alternative Medicine section of this book.

Suffice it to say, that numerous people ascribe their recovery from cancer to vitamin B17 and it is widely recommended by practitioners of alternative medicine.

The mode of action is based upon the fact that each molecule of vitamin B17 contains one unit of hydrogen cyanide, one unit of benzaldehyde and two units of glucose tightly locked together.

The cyanide molecule can only become dangerous if the entire B17 molecule is dismantled.

Fortunately, we lack the enzymes necessary to break the molecule down, which makes it harmless to healthy tissue. Cancer cells, however, contain the necessary enzyme called beta-glucosidase. That means that when vitamin B17 disperses throughout your body, it is only broken down into cyanide within cancer cells, thereby creating a targeted therapy.

However, mainstream medicine / the pharmaceutical industry do not concur with the research, which is unsurprising considering that if vitamin B17 were proven to be effective in the treatment of cancer, it would entirely undermine $200 billion per year in revenues. In my honest opinion, I believe it worthy of significant impartial research.

I now eat the seeds of my apples.

Apricots

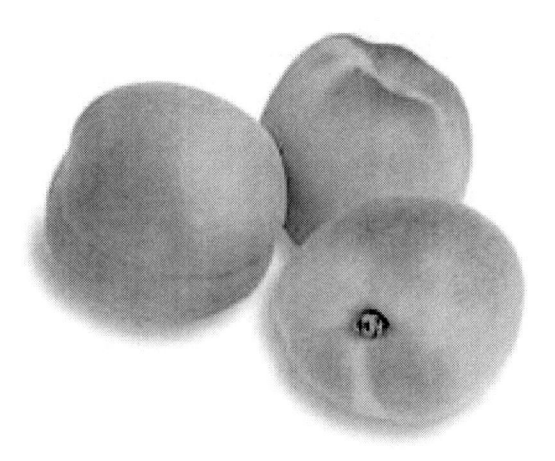

Apricots are an excellent source of vitamin A and beta-carotene, along with vitamin C, fibre, quercetin and lycopene which all exhibit cancer fighting properties. In a dried form, they make excellent healthy snacks. The American Cancer Society states that apricots and other foods that are rich in carotenes have the potential to lower the risk of various cancers, including those of the oesophagus, lungs and larynx.

A study of over 50,000 registered female nurses also discovered that those nurses consuming the highest quantities of vitamin A, reduced the likelihood of developing cataracts by nearly 40%, making apricots a fantastic preserver of eye health, by preventing free radical damage to eye tissues over time.

The dried apricots you might get from your supermarket are a bright orange colour, but naturally, apricots turn brown after a short period of time. Maintaining this bright orange colour is due to treatment by sulphur dioxide, which is a preserving agent. Health food stores normally provide unprocessed apricots, which are brown but taste the same.

The seed within the apricots contain significant quantities of vitamin B17, which as described in the preceding section on Apples, has been cited as being one of the most important tools against cancer by many practitioners of alternative medicine.

You can purchase apricots seeds from health food stores, although they may be more difficult to acquire in certain countries.

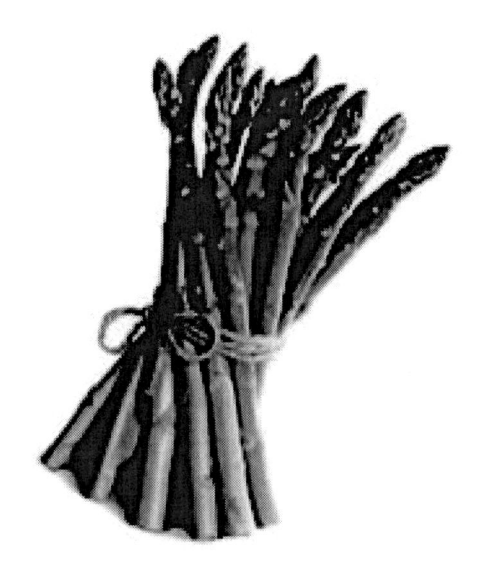

Asparagus

Asparagus is a great source of vitamin C, vitamin B6, and thiamine. It also contains rutin, which is a flavonoid that is thought to possess anti-inflammatory properties. It strengthens blood vessels and can protect against oxidative tissue damage. Asparagus is also high in glutathione, which is an antioxidant that helps protect against free radicals.

Another plant chemical found in Asparagus, protodioscin, has been linked to the reduction of bone loss, an increase in sexual desire and studies have indicated that it can have an impact on several different forms of cancer cells.

It is an excellent source of folic acid, which has been shown to help control your levels of homocysteine. When folate levels are low, blood levels of homocysteine may rise, which can significantly increase your risk for heart disease and atherosclerosis.

Where diabetes is concerned, a 2006 study reported in the British Journal of Medicine, showed that an extract of Asparagus was able to improve the action of insulin, creating an 81% increase in the glucose uptake of fat cells. This is important because it would help to lower blood sugar levels, and an excess of blood sugar promotes premature ageing and damage to almost all of our issues.

In terms of digestive health, Asparagus contains inulin, which is a carbohydrate that isn't easily digested, but does provide a food source for the friendly bacteria in our gut, helping to promote the bacteria that improve our digestion and strengthen our immune system.

Overall, asparagus is an excellent addition to your diet, even if it is less frequent than some of the other fruit and vegetables recommended in this guide.

Avocados

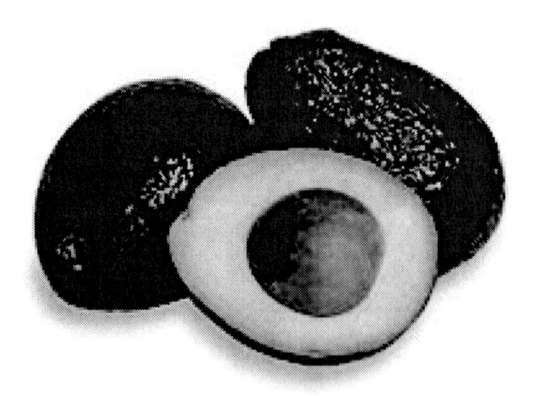

A study conducted by the UCLA Centre for Human Nutrition showed that when avocado extract was added to prostate cancer cells, cell growth was inhibited by up to 60%.

Aside from the UCLA study data, avocados are one of the rare fruit that contain an excellent source of healthy fat. They are fantastic as part of a salad, because the fat within the avocado greatly increases your body's ability to absorb the nutrition in the rest of your food.

Many nutrients require fat to transport them into the body, which is the biggest problem with low-fat diets that can leave you malnourished. Eating avocado in combination with other fruit and vegetables, has been shown to increase your absorption of lutein four times over, your absorption of alpha-carotene, eight times over, and boost your absorption of beta-carotene, a whopping 13 times over! Beta-carotene has excellent anti-cancer properties, so being able to increase its absorption is very important.

Avocados are also rich in the amino acid tryptophan, with a side order of vitamin B6 and folic acid. These key nutrients are used in the synthesis of serotonin, which is the feel-good neurotransmitter in your brain. Serotonin is vitally important when it comes to elevating your mood and fending off depression. As you will see in the psychology section of this book, your mood can have a drastic impact upon survival rates, so never underestimate the value of looking after your emotional health.

Finally, avocado contains natural antibiotic and antifungal chemicals.

Bananas

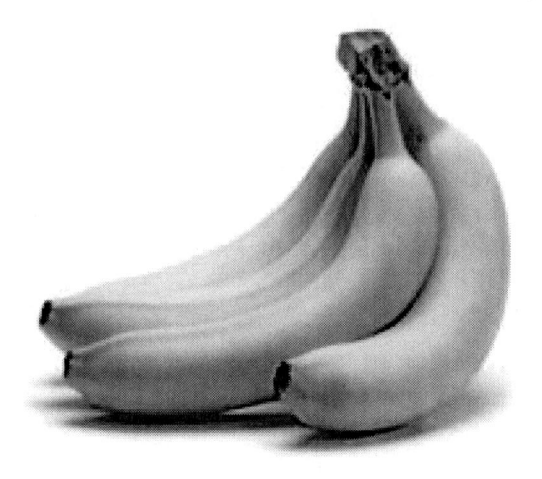

Bananas are an excellent source of vitamin C, vitamin B6, and fibre. Green bananas are also a source of resistant starch, which is digested more slowly and does not cause blood sugar to surge. It is believed that resistant starch could reduce the risk of a number of different types of cancer, including colon cancer.

Certainly in the case of kidney cancer, a large population study discovered that women who consumed bananas around 4 to 6 times per week reduced their risk of kidney cancer by up to 50% compared with women who didn't eat bananas at all.

Barley

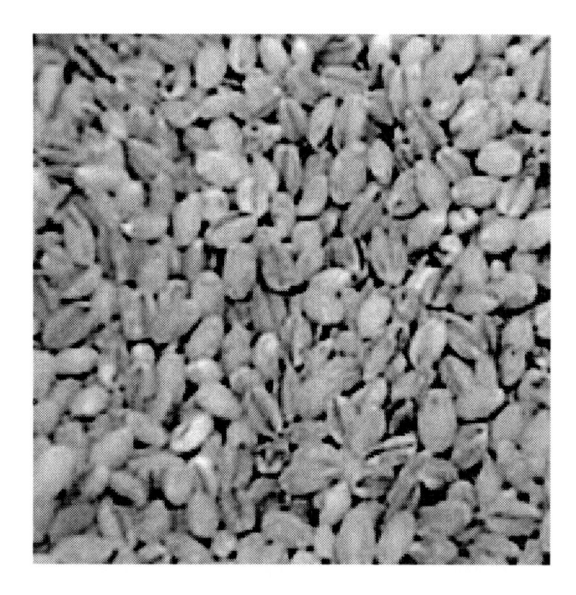

Barley is an excellent source of both soluble and insoluble fibre. Two different rat studies have indicated significant benefits from consuming Barley in your diet. The first, demonstrated that Barley increases bowel movement and relieves constipation (which reduces your risk of bowel cancer), and the second showed that in rats with existing colon cancer, the group fed on Barley had significantly fewer tumours than the other groups.

This could be due to the effects of the fibre enabling the colon to function correctly, or it could be due to a number of the other anti-cancer compounds found within the Barley including beta-glucans, which aid in immune function and help to lower cholesterol. Other antioxidants, including selenium, quercetin and phenolic acids have all been shown to help reduce cell damage from free radicals, and exert an anti-cancer effect.

To include Barley in your diet, you can replace anywhere up to 50% of the wheat flour you use with Barley flour (although I would advocate you eliminate wheat from your diet altogether if possible), or else you can add cooked Barley to other foods such as soups and salads. Barley flakes are a very simple addition to breakfast cereal.

Beans

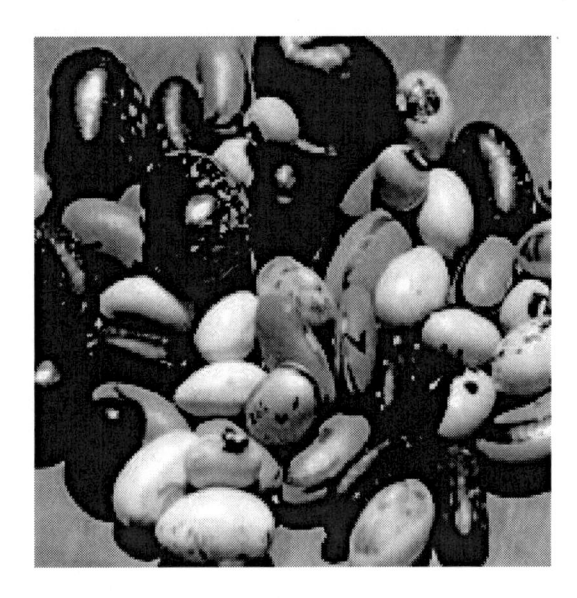

Beans and other pulses, are digested slowly by the body to give a sustained release of energy. This helps to moderate blood sugar levels which is a good way of slowing the ageing process. Much of the way our tissues age is due to glycation from the excess blood sugar we get from high carbohydrate food sources.

Eating beans and other pulses also helps to stimulate the production of hyaluronic acid which is a substance that occurs naturally in the skin. Hyaluronic acid helps your skin to retain water within the skin cells, basically acting as a moisturiser that keeps your skin smooth and wrinkle free. Of course collagen and elastin play their part but a good intake of vitamin C and vitamin E in fruit and nuts covers that requirement. The important thing is that levels of hyaluronic acid decrease as your skin ages.

Most importantly where cancer is concerned, is that in addition to the other phytonutrients, and protein, beans provide high levels of dietary fibre which can help keep bowel movements more regular and lowers your risk of colorectal cancer.

Studies have also indicated a reduction in breast cancer risk in postmenopausal women associated with the consumption of beans.

Beetroot, or beets

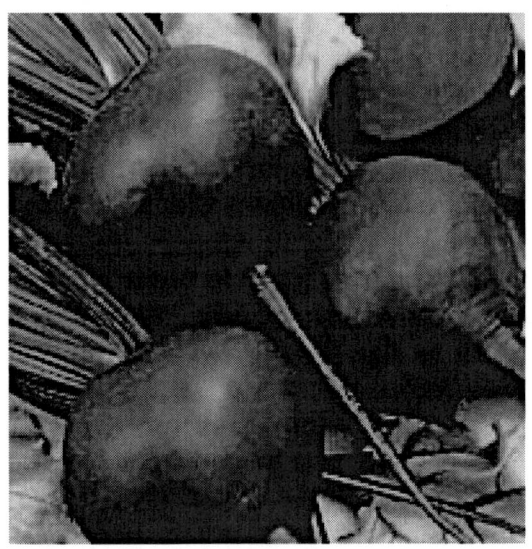

Beetroot contains a whole range of active ingredients that can help to fight cancer. Firstly, the red pigment (betacyanin) found in beetroot has some anticarcinogenic properties, but not only that, beets also have the property of being able to increase the cellular intake of oxygen by as much as 400%.

This is great news, because cancer cells respond very poorly to elevated levels of oxygen. In fact, a recent study revealed that beetroot juice enabled people to exercise for up to 16% longer because they required less oxygen for the same level of aerobic activity!

Beets also contain manganese, which is needed for your body's production of interferon, which has been shown in studies to act as a powerful anti-cancer agent.

In addition, betaine, found in beetroot, stimulates liver cells to eliminate toxins. This defence of the liver and bile ducts enables your liver to function more effectively, which detoxifies your whole system.

Many cancer patients have a heavy load placed upon their livers, so any mechanism to improve the function is a good idea. Beetroot juice not only contains high levels of betaine, but it is also alkaline which helps reverse acidosis, which is a precursor for a number of diseases. Any foods that encourage an alkaline environment set up a hostile environment for cancer, because cancer cells prefer acidic conditions within the body.

Beetroot juice has also been found to widen blood vessels, which reduces blood pressure. Just a single 250ml glass each day was clinically proven to significantly lower blood pressure just 24 hours later. Researchers discovered that the active ingredient that achieves this effect was nitrates, because nitrates formed nitric oxide in the blood. They also found that taking nitrates in tablet form achieved the same effect.

Finally, beetroot juice can also combat the effects of nitrites, (not to be confused with nitrates) which are the chemical preservatives used in cured meat products, such as ham. Nitrites have been shown to increase your risk of stomach and bowel cancer. Better to avoid nitrites in cured meats altogether, but if you don't, then try to consume them with beetroot on the side (as part of a salad) or as beetroot juice.

One word of warning though, for anyone that has not consumed much beetroot before, not everybody has the enzymes necessary to break down the coloured pigment, so you may experience purple or red urine, which is known as beeturia. But this is perfectly harmless.

Berries

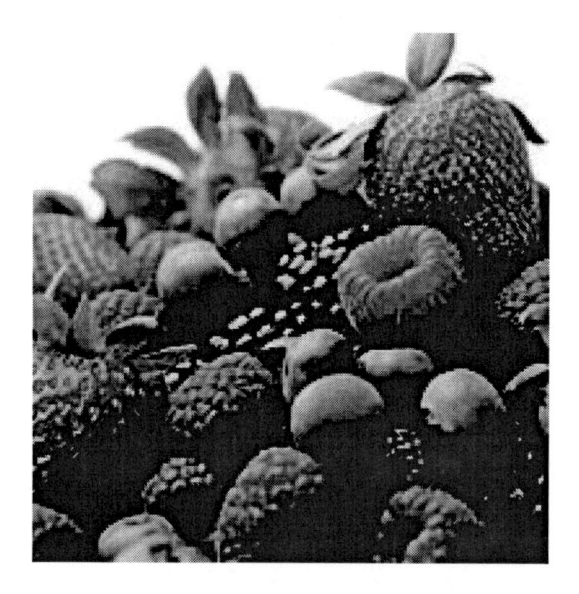

Please see blackberries, blueberries, cranberries, raspberries, and strawberries.

Blackberries

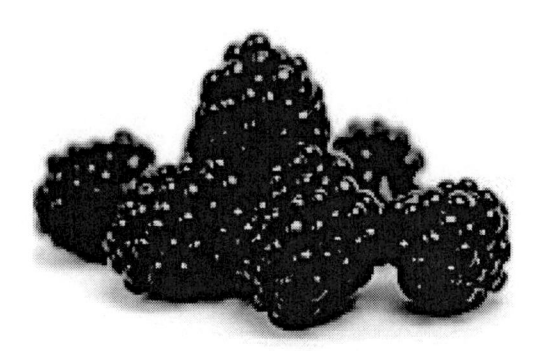

Blackberries are an excellent source of antioxidants which help to mop up the free radicals within our bodies. This prevents the free radicals from then causing damage to your body's tissues - particularly in the liver and colon. Studies show that blackberries have a higher antioxidant capacity than cranberries, strawberries, raspberries and even blueberries.

They contain fibre, vitamin C, vitamin E, ellagic acid and the phytochemicals cyanidin, tannin and flavonoid. All of which have been shown to be anticarcinogenic.

Another active ingredient is quercetin, a form of catechin which has been shown to act as an antioxidant that can reduce the risk of heart disease and reduce allergic reactions. In lab rats, blackberries were shown to reduce the growth rates of oesophageal cancer.

Studies conducted on human lung cancer cells demonstrated that a blackberry extract (anthocyanin) inhibited further cancer growth, and this was reinforced by laboratory studies on rats that showed inhibited tumour promotion and metastasis (the spread of cancer cells). Blackberries really are a superfood where cancer is concerned.

Blueberries

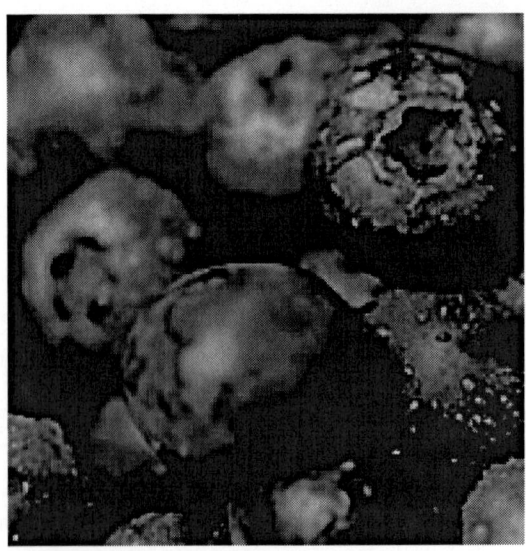

High in antioxidants, blueberries are excellent for detoxifying the body and providing protection against free radicals caused by stress, smoking, poor diet and a range of other factors. Studies also suggest that the dark pigments contained within blueberries, known as anthocyanins, may protect against diseases like Parkinson's, Alzheimer's and other neurodegenerative diseases.

Interestingly, memory experts, including the US grand champion, Ronnie White, highly recommend blueberries as a part of your diet if you intend to compete in memory tournaments.

Many of the compounds within blueberries are also found in blackberries, so please also see the Blackberry section.

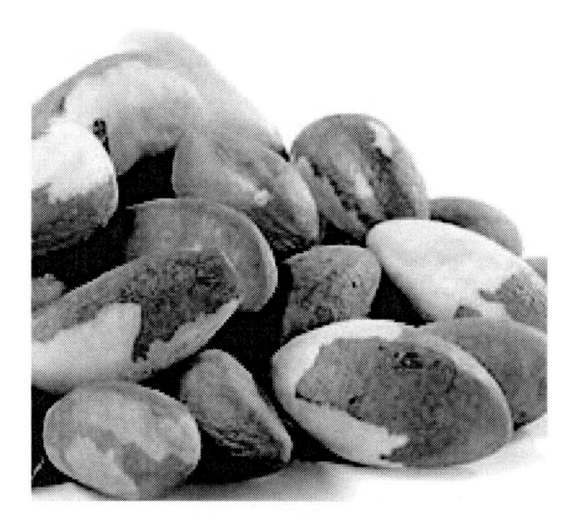

Brazil Nuts

Brazil nuts have been found to be more protective against cancer than pure selenium selenite. They contain an abundance of selenium, which is a mineral that has mood boosting properties, which can include relieving fatigue, anxiety and depression. They also contain ellagic acid, a compound that blocks enzymes that are necessary for the growth of cancer cells.

Combine that with the enzyme glutathione, (which suppresses free radicals and has been shown in studies to slow or halt the development of tumours), vitamin E, magnesium, iron and omega-6 essential fatty acids and you have probably the most nutritious nut of them all. You should try to eat some everyday, along with walnuts and almonds.

Power Combination: combine Brazil nuts with cabbage or broccoli or other sources of sulforaphane such as watercress, or rocket. According to the Institute of Food Research, if you combine sulforaphane with selenium (in Brazil nuts), the combined cancer fighting properties are up to 13 times more potent than either one alone. You also get selenium in walnuts, eggs, soya beans and seafood. Try adding chopped Brazil nuts to coleslaw or sauerkraut, or a grating them onto a rocket salad.

Broccoli

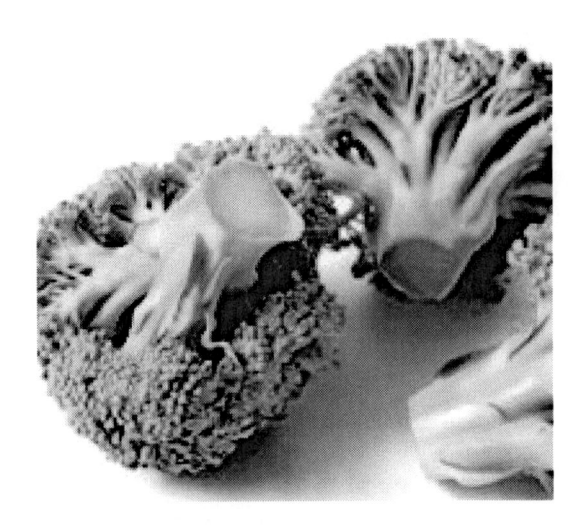

Much interest in cancer prevention is focused on cruciferous vegetables like broccoli, cabbage, and cauliflower. Broccoli contains indoles, including sulphuraphane, an isothiocyanate that seems to inhibit breast tumours.

Broccoli also contains glucosinolates, which, when consumed along with the necessary enzyme to break them down (which is in the broccoli itself) , have been shown to reduce the risk of prostate, breast, lung and colorectal cancer.

By weight, fresh broccoli, boiled and drained, has 16% more vitamin C than an orange, roughly as much calcium as milk, a significant amount of iron, and the stalk is high in fibre.

Power Combination: combine broccoli with Brazil nuts or walnuts, eggs, soya beans or seafood because the addition of selenium greatly increases the cancer fighting properties of the broccoli.

Power Combination: combine broccoli with tomatoes. Tomatoes are a potent source of lycopene. When lycopene was combined with the glycosinolates in broccoli, animal studies showed a tomato/broccoli combination was able to reduce tumour size by up to 52%. Be sure to include a little bit of cold-pressed olive oil, to help with the digestion of lycopene because it is fat-soluble and needs the oil to help your body absorb it.

Cabbage

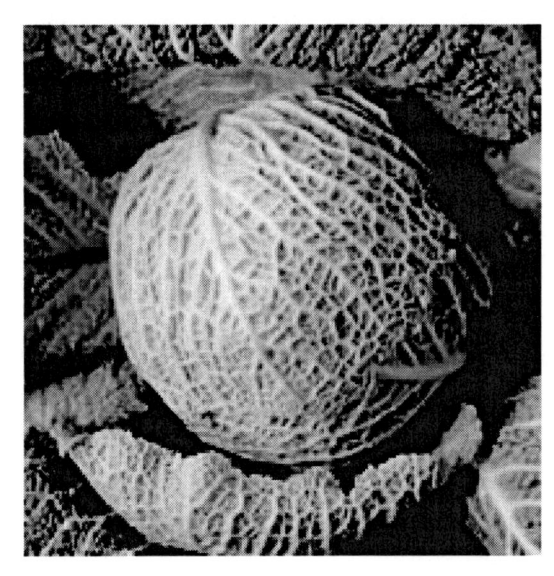

A study published in the journal Cancer Prevention Research in 2010 highlighted an exciting new benefit to consuming cabbage, broccoli, brussels sprouts, cauliflower and other cruciferous vegetables.

Consuming these vegetables encourages your body to synthesise indole-3-carbinol. This substance, otherwise known as I3C helps to break down a protein complex that is associated with excessive and deregulated reproduction of cells.

The protein complex known as Cdc25A, has been shown to be significantly elevated in cases of breast cancer, lung cancer, prostate cancer and cancers of the head and neck, liver, oesophagus, endometrium and colon. Typically, the higher the level of Cdc25A, the poorer the prognosis for the patient.

If the hallmark of cancer is the uncontrolled and deregulated reproduction of cells caused by the excess Cdc25A, and the I3C helps to prevent this, (and therefore helps to stop the spread / growth of cancer) then it makes cruciferous vegetables, including cabbage, a vital feature of any anti-cancer diet.

The researchers went on to say "Cdc25A is present at abnormally high levels in about half of breast cancer cases, and it is associated with a poor prognosis".

"I3C can have striking effects on cancer cells, and a better understanding of this mechanism may lead to the use of this dietary supplement as an effective and safe strategy for treating a variety of cancers and other human diseases associated with the over-expression of Cdc25A."

In the laboratory, when researchers exposed cultured breast cancer cells to I3C, they discovered that it destroyed the excess Cdc25A. They then moved on to animal trials, where they were able to demonstrate that dietary supplements containing active ingredients from broccoli and brussels sprouts were able to reduce the breast cancer tumour sizes in mice by up to 65% when administered orally.

Cabbage contains glucosinolates, isothiocyanates, vitamin C and dietary fibre, all of which have been shown to exert an anti-cancer effect, slowing or preventing the growth of cancer cells.

Cabbage can be added to your diet in a number of ways, from being included in salad, being boiled or steamed and added to a roast dinner, all the way through to being fermented and eaten as sauerkraut.

A Polish women's health study conducted upon hundreds of Polish and Polish-born women (now living in the US), revealed that the women who consumed three or more servings of cabbage per week were 72% less likely to develop breast cancer in comparison with their counterparts, who only consumed one and a half servings per week or less. The portions included raw, lightly cooked or fermented cabbage in the form of sauerkraut.

Carrots

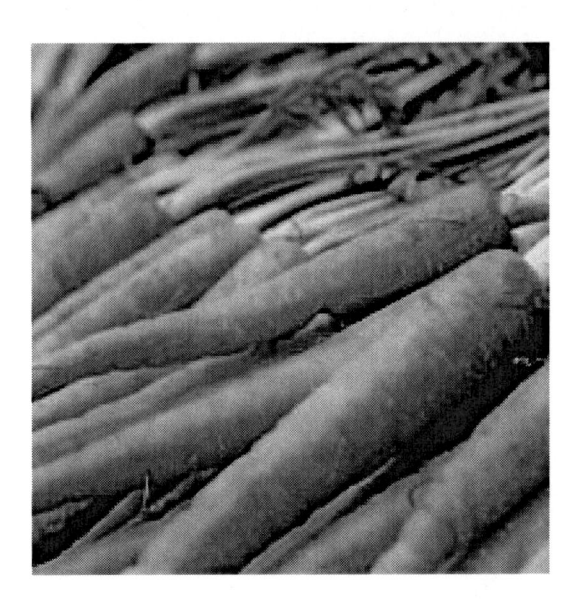

Carrots contain a class of fat-soluble pigments called carotenoids. These carotenoids can vary in colour from yellow to orange to red. They protect cells from the damaging effects of free radicals and enhance the functioning of the immune system by increasing the number of white blood cells in the immune system, including T cells.

The most common carotenoids are beta-carotene, lycopene, lutein, beta-crpytoxanthin, zeaxanthin, and astaxanthin, and can be found in other fruit and vegetables such as sweet potatoes, kale, tomatoes, spinach, red peppers and apricots.

Eating these foods raw, or lightly steaming them will help to retain the carotenoids. It is also important that they are eaten with a certain amount of oil, perhaps a drizzle of cold-pressed olive oil, to ensure that they are adequately absorbed through the gut. This is because the carotenoids are fat-soluble.

There have been multiple studies showing that carotenoids substantially reduce the risk of breast cancer. In a study of 5,450 postmenopausal women studied over an eight-year period, (published in the International Journal of Cancer 2009), higher consumption of carotenoid laden vegetables almost cut their risk of invasive breast cancer in half.

In another study, (published in Cancer Epidemiology, Biomarkers and Prevention, 2009), which looked into women with all different stages of breast cancer, (from the earliest stages right up until recurrence of the disease after previously successful treatment), the study concluded that "higher biological exposure to carotenoids, when assessed over the time frame of the study, was associated with greater likelihood of breast cancer-free survival, regardless of study group assignment."

Of course, the studies presented here relate to breast cancer, but that does not mean that carotenoids do not have an effect on other forms of cancer, or their prevention.

Power Combination: combine any sources of beta-carotene with avocado, because the fat in avocado has been shown to increase the absorption of beta-carotene by up to 13 times over. Alternatively, a drizzle of cold-pressed olive oil will help too.

Cauliflower

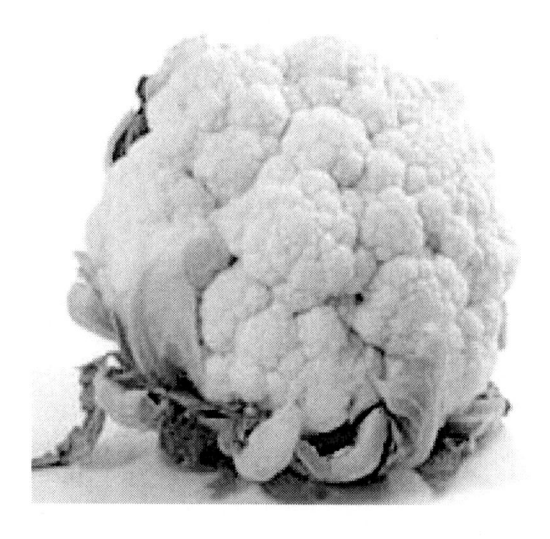

As you will have seen in the cabbage section, compounds within cauliflower stimulate the production of I3C, which suppresses the protein that triggers excessive cell reproduction that is common to many types of cancer.

Like broccoli, cauliflower also contains indoles, including sulphuraphane, an isothiocyanate that seems to inhibit breast tumours.

Cauliflower also contains glucosinolates, which have been shown in studies to decrease the risk of prostate, breast, lung and colorectal cancer.

Celery

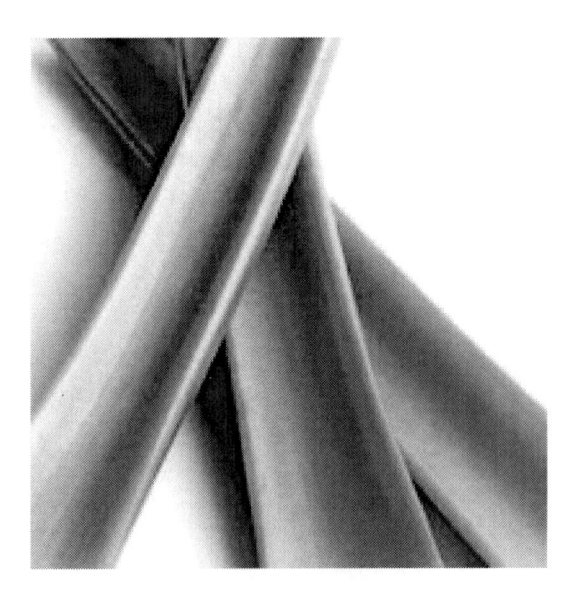

Celery contains a number of nutrients. It is high in vitamin A and contains vitamin C, vitamin B1, vitamin B2, calcium, iron, magnesium, phosphorus and potassium.

In animal studies, celery juice has been shown to significantly lower cholesterol by increasing the production of bile acid.

With regard to cancer, a significant substance found within the essential oil of celery seeds is perillyl alcohol. Animal studies have yielded significant results, indicating the usefulness of perillyl alcohol in regressing pancreatic, stomach, colon, skin, mammary and liver tumours. The strength of this research has prompted the National Cancer Institute to conduct human (phase II) clinical trials to determine the effectiveness of perillyl alcohol in halting breast cancer.

Perillyl alcohol can be isolated from the essential oils of several plants including cherries, lavender, peppermint, spearmint, celery seeds, sage, cranberries, lemongrass, ginger grass, savin juniper, Conyza newii, caraway, Perilla frutescens, and wild bergamont.

Cheese

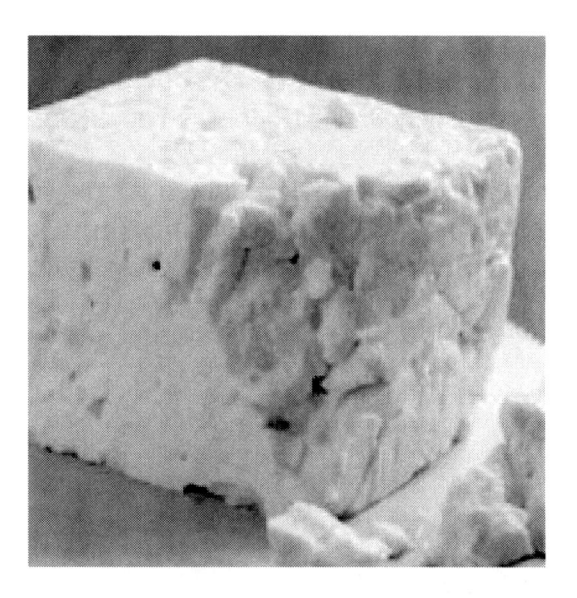

Whilst there are some question marks surrounding dairy products in relation to cancer, several notable studies have been published indicating the extraordinary benefits of vitamin K2 which is found in high concentrations in fermented or mature cheeses. Blue cheeses, feta cheese, or aged hard cheeses such as mature cheddar are all high in vitamin K2, otherwise known as menaquinone.

Vitamin K1, can be derived from a number of vegetable sources, but it is the vitamin K2 that has been shown to be so extraordinarily effective in preventing cancer.

Vitamin K2 can also be found at lower levels in chicken, beef, liver, some animal fats and sauerkraut.

In a study published in the American Journal of Clinical Nutrition 2010, which analysed data from over 24,000 participants covering a ten-year period, the researchers discovered that those who consumed the greatest levels of vitamin K2 were 14% less likely to develop cancer, and 28% less likely to die of it, in comparison with those who had the lowest intake.

In another study, conducted by researchers at the Mayo Clinic, it was discovered that individuals with the highest levels of dietary vitamin K2 intake had a 45% lower risk of developing a cancer of the immune system called non-Hodgkin's lymphoma.

Other research has also shown that vitamin K2 can be a beneficial factor in preventing or reducing additional forms of cancer including cancer of the liver, stomach, colon and mouth.

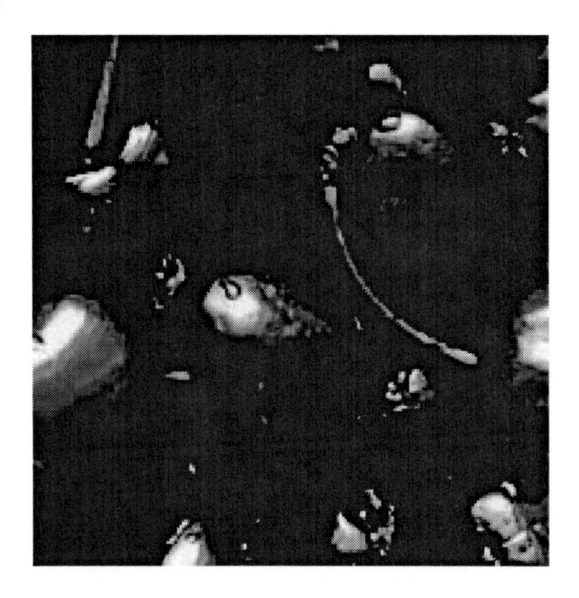

Cherries

Cherries contain vitamin A, a range of B vitamins, vitamin C, calcium, potassium, iron and dietary fibre, making them a healthy choice provided that they are organic. Unfortunately, cherries were listed in the top 12 foods to be most contaminated with pesticides by the Environmental Working Group, a consumer advocate and research organisation, so buying organic is important.

Cherries are loaded with anti-inflammatory, anti-ageing and anti-cancer compounds, including perillyl alcohol (see Celery), ellagic acid (which kills cancer cells in the lab, with no change to healthy, normal cells), anthocyanins and quercetin (which not only have anti-cancer properties, but also help relieve the effects of allergies and inflammation).

In the case of diabetes, the anthocyanins in tart cherries have been found to increase the production of insulin in animal pancreatic cells by as much as 50%.

Chili Peppers

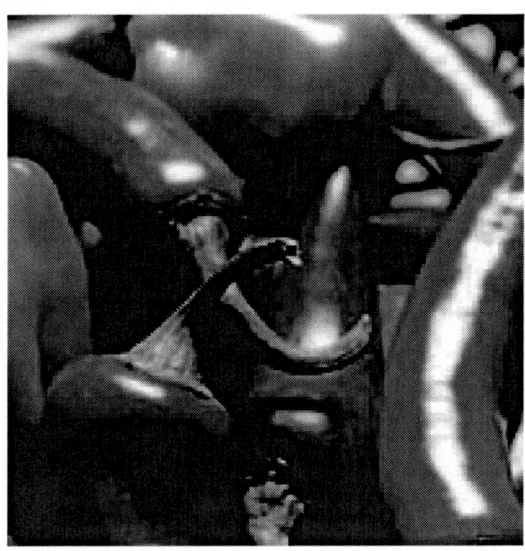

Capsaicin, the active ingredient in chilli peppers that makes them "hot", has a number of anti-cancer, anti-inflammatory and heart-health boosting properties.

A study conducted at Nottingham University in the UK showed that Capsaicin killed laboratory cultured lung cancer cells and pancreatic cancer cells, by attacking the cells' source of energy and triggering programmed cell death. Furthermore, the capsaicin did this without harming the surrounding tissue.

Dr. Timothy Bates, who led the study, reported "This is incredibly exciting and may explain why people living in countries like Mexico and India, who traditionally eat a diet which is very spicy, tend to have lower incidences of many cancers that are prevalent in the Western world."

"We appear to have discovered a fundamental weakness with all cancer cells. Capsaicin specifically targets cancerous cells, leading to the possibility that a drug based on it would kill tumors with few or no side effects for the patient."

Researchers from the University of Cincinnati also discovered that they could significantly reduce the damage to heart cells during a heart attack if they applied a topical cream containing capsaicin to the skin, because it triggered certain nervous system responses and "pro-survival pathways" that protect the heart. In animal studies, the scientists discovered an incredible 85% reduction in heart cell death when they used the cream, which makes it the most powerful cardioprotective substance detected so far.

Capsaicin is already used in a number of topical medications for pain relief.

It appears that habanero peppers have the highest levels of capsaicin of any pepper, and in mouse studies conducted by UCLA in 2009, researchers were able to shrink prostate tumours by 80%, verses untreated mice. This was done over a 2 month period, using the human equivalent of 8 fresh habanero peppers, (or 400mg capsaicin), eaten 3 times per week for a 170lb man.

Research conducted at the University of Pittsburgh Medical School showed that capsaicin induced apoptosis (programmed cell death) in pancreatic cancer cells.

More recent research has shown that capsaicin has inhibited the growth of adult leukaemia cells and gastric cancer.

Chocolate

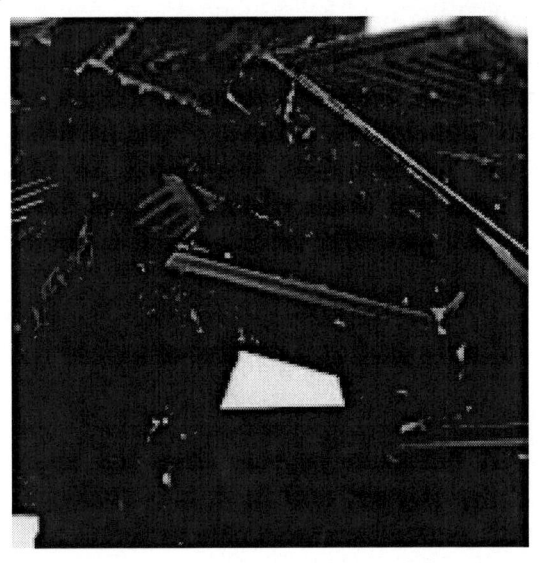

Dark chocolate is a rich source of antioxidants. In fact it has a number of health benefits. Chocolate comes from cocoa beans, which contain more flavonols and polyphenols than many other fruit and vegetables. It also contains calcium, iron, zinc and magnesium making it helpful for maintaining your immune system and strong, healthy bones and teeth.

In the form of dark chocolate or cocoa powder, there is more antioxidant capacity than in many fruit juices. However, hot chocolate, due to the alkalisation process, contains little, if any.

Numerous studies have shown that the flavanols in chocolate lower blood pressure, reducing the risk of heart disease, blood clots and strokes, compared with individuals who do not eat chocolate. One particular study showed that people who ate chocolate once per week, were 22% less likely to have a stroke than people who ate no chocolate. A second study found that people who ate 50g of chocolate once per week, were 46% less likely to die following a stroke than people who didn't eat chocolate at all.

A German study published in the European Heart Journal showed that those people who averaged at least 7.5g per day of chocolate were nearly 40% less likely to have a heart attack, compared with those who ate only 1.7g per day on average. Just having a single square of chocolate per day can make all the difference!

The main thing is to avoid drastically increasing your calorie intake, and the closer the chocolate is to unrefined pure cocoa, the better. Try to opt for the chocolate that is 70% or greater cocoa. Processing the chocolate to sweeten it, such as in the case of milk chocolate or white chocolate, substantially reduces its effectiveness.

Citrus fruit

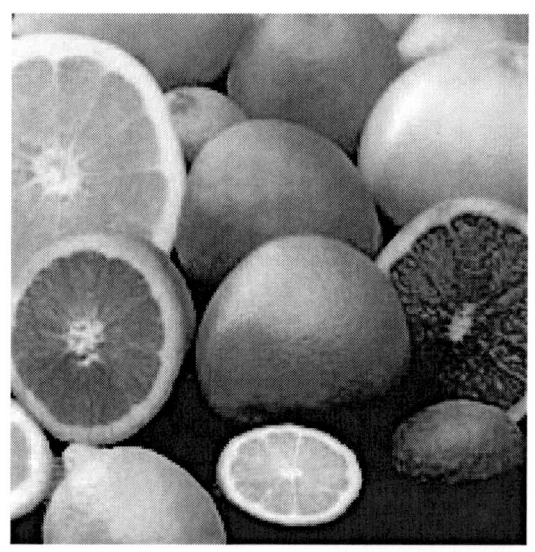

Citrus fruits contain chemicals called monoterpenes, including d-limonene. Such chemicals have shown particular value in preventing breast, liver and lung cancer. Eating these fruits will help boost your cancer fighting ability, although there are greater concentrations of the helpful chemicals in the peel of the fruit.

A new study from Japan (published in the International Journal of Cancer) indicates that daily consumption of citrus fruit may reduce risk of a range of different cancers, including pancreatic and prostate cancer. The study averaged an 11 to 14% reduction in the incidence of all types of cancer for both men and women that consumed citrus fruit daily, but this rate was improved upon by the addition of a cup of green tea each day.

The data from this study was significant because it covered over 42,000 people over a nine-year period. The average age of the study participants was 59 years old.

Please also see the sections on Oranges, Lemons and Grapefruit.

Coconut oil.

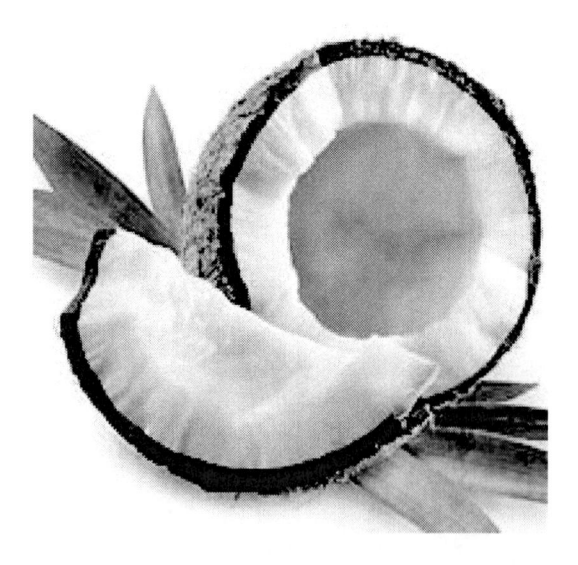

Although Coconut oil is a saturated fat, not all saturated fats are bad. In fact, half of the fat content of Coconut oil is a rare form of fat called lauric acid. It has unique health promoting properties, in particular the fact that it is antibacterial, anti-viral, antifungal and anti-protozoa.

It also has properties that help it contribute toward weight loss (which in itself reduces your risk of cancer), as it speeds up your metabolism and enables you to burn more calories in a day.

A recent study, published in the journal Lipids in 2009, showed that a group of women supplemented with 30ml of Coconut oil per day had a significant reduction in their waist circumference compared with the control group.

The circumference of your waist is a measure of abdominal obesity, which is a key indicator associated with heart disease and type II diabetes. This indicated that Coconut oil could help in both of these conditions, but further tests also showed that those consuming Coconut oil raised their healthy HDL cholesterol levels and lowered their LDL to HDL cholesterol ratio, which should reduce their risk of cardiovascular disease.

Most importantly, Coconut oil is excellent for cooking with because it does not sustain a great deal of heat damage when you cook with it. This means less free radicals consumed with your food. You should use it when you are frying or baking, or else you can literally just consume it each day as part of a hot drink or on its own.

Saturated fats such as coconut oil also do not hinder the body's ability to utilise vitamin D, which can be a problem with polyunsaturated fats. Vitamin D has excellent anti-cancer properties, and deficiencies in it are linked with a whole host of age-related illnesses. Please see the Fish section for more information on this.

Cranberries

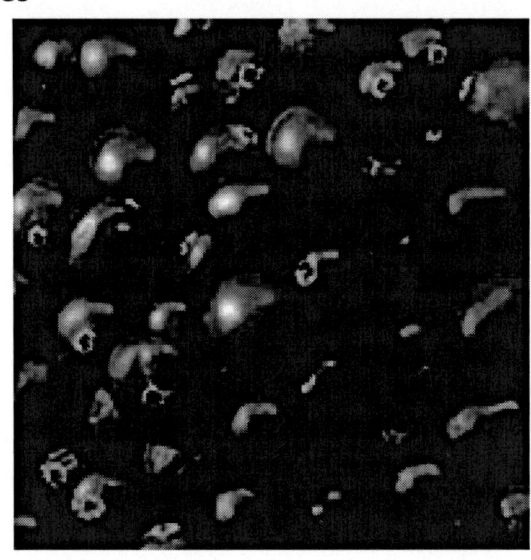

According to a study published in the Journal of Agricultural and Food Chemistry, Cranberries contain more phenolic antioxidants than 19 of the most popular fruits. They are packed with vitamin C, fibre and a range of other phytonutrients.

A number of studies have confirmed that the flavonoids within Cranberries have an impact upon your body's ability to fight breast cancer, lung cancer, colorectal cancer, leukaemia and potentially a number of other forms of cancer.

The same compounds may also reduce the risk of atherosclerosis and heart disease, because they reduce the LDL (bad) cholesterol and potentially raise levels of HDL (good) cholesterol.

Interestingly, it seems as though cranberry juice may be just as effective, so it is an easy option to add this to your diet. Just be sure to have juice that doesn't contain added sugar. The unsweetened juice can be a little bitter, but you can mix it with apple juice to improve the flavour. Alternatively, you can add the berries to your breakfast or salads.

Cruciferous vegetables

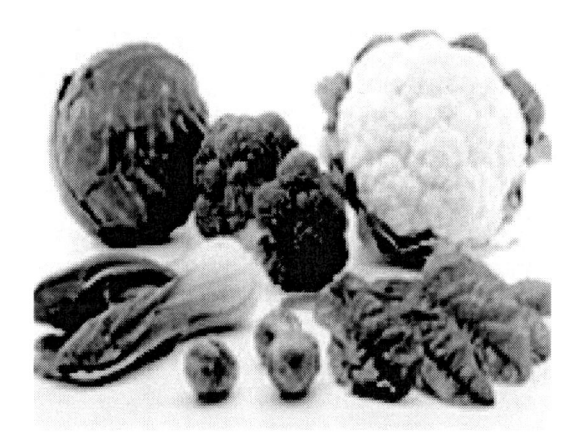

Cruciferous vegetables contain high levels of glucosinolates, which have been shown to reduce the likelihood of prostate, lung, breast and colorectal cancer. However, glucosinolates can only be utilised by the body if you also consume the necessary enzyme that breaks them down.

The enzyme, called myrosinase, is present in the actual raw vegetable, so all you have to do is to consume it without cooking it to excess. Cooking these vegetables until they are soft and mushy can reduce your intake of these valuable cancer fighting compounds by as much as eight times. Lightly cooking for just two to three minutes, or lightly steaming allows you to retain adequate levels of the enzyme.

The hydrolysis product of glucosinolates are isothiocyanates. These compounds help us to detoxify by increasing the action of detoxification enzymes, they prevent oxidative DNA and cell damage and in numerous studies have been shown to reduce the incidence and rate of chemically induced mammary tumours in animals, and inhibit the growth of cultured human breast cancer cells, leading to cell death.

In one study of 1000 men, it revealed that those men who consumed three or more servings of cruciferous vegetables per week had a 41% reduction in their risk of prostate cancer compared with those that only consumed one or less portion per week.

If you aren't a fan of broccoli, cabbage and cauliflower, you can also consider kale, brussels sprouts, watercress, Oriental cabbage, radish, wassabi and various mustards.

Please also see the sections on Broccoli, Cabbage, and Cauliflower to discover their unique individual properties.

Dark green leafy vegetables

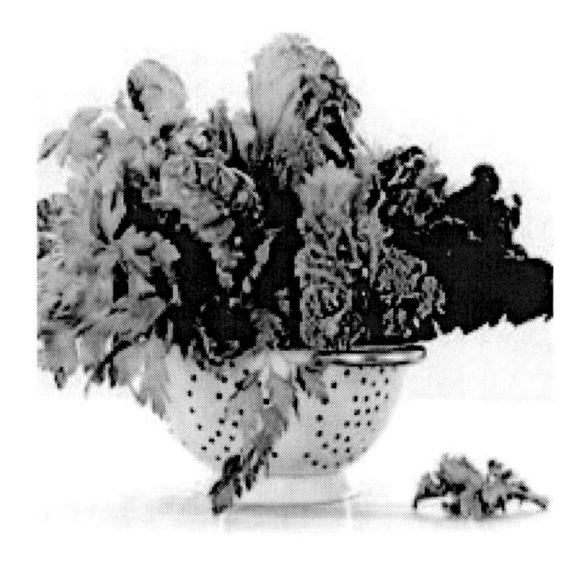

Numerous studies consistently confirm that the consumption of green leafy vegetables greatly reduce our risk of both heart disease and cancer.

Such vegetables include spinach, kale, watercress, lettuce, rocket, parsley, wheatgrass and chicory.

In addition to the vitamins, minerals and fat burning compounds they contain, they are also rich in chlorophyll. This is the green pigment within the plant that enables it to convert energy from the sun.

The important thing is that because chlorophyll is structurally similar to the haemoglobin in our blood, studies have shown that an increased consumption of chlorophyll has resulted in greater production of haemoglobin within the blood. Haemoglobin is how our blood cells transport oxygen around our bodies.

Numerous studies have shown that cancer cells respond very poorly to increased levels of oxygen, so it stands to reason that if you increase your haemoglobin levels, your body is becoming a more hostile environment for cancer cells.

Eggs (Free Range and preferably organic).

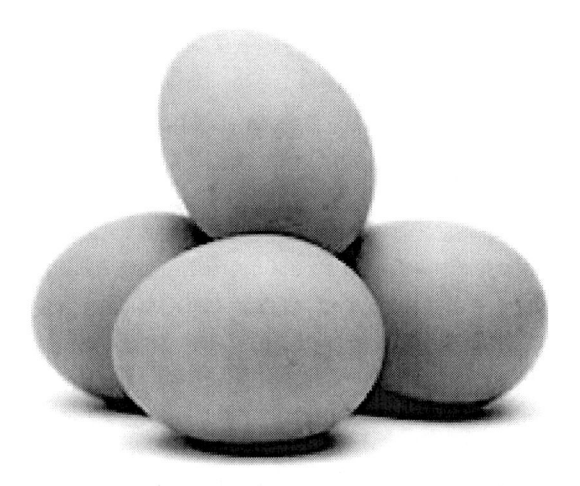

Eggs are an economical way to get some fantastic nutrition into your diet. However, as I mentioned in the Introduction of this book, not all eggs are created equal. For best results, make sure that you are consuming free range eggs, preferably organic and certainly not processed battery hen eggs.

In addition to the omega-3 and omega-6 essential fatty acids, eggs also contain nine different essential amino acids, making them one of the best sources of protein available. Quality protein is vital in the production of your hormones, operating your immune system and the general repair of your body.

Eggs also contain zeaxanthin and lutein for healthy eyes along with vitamin B12 and choline, which supports your heart, nervous system and brain.

Some people have seen the mainstream media assertion that eggs are bad for you because of the cholesterol. The fact is, the bulk of the cholesterol in your body is created when you have an excess of blood sugar. It is not down to the amount of cholesterol you consume in your diet.

The cholesterol in eggs is just a tiny amount in comparison with the level of cholesterol you have in your bloodstream at any one time.

If you have high levels of cholesterol, you should not cut down your consumption of nutritious eggs, you should cut down your consumption of nutritionally empty carbohydrates, in particular those derived from wheat, and processed sugar.

Egg yolk contains the amino acids tryptophan and tyrosine, which have been proven to exert antioxidant effects. In fact, a single raw egg yolk has the same antioxidant capacity as an Apple. The antioxidant properties are reduced by about half when boiled or fried, but nevertheless they are still very biologically active when cooked.

Previous studies have also shown that when egg proteins are converted by enzymes in the stomach and small intestine, they produce peptides that act within the body the same way as ACE inhibitors, which are prescription drugs used to reduce blood pressure. This contradicts the mainstream media portrayal of eggs being bad for blood pressure due to the cholesterol present within them.

In the interests of getting a balanced diet however, I recommend that you should not consume more than 2 eggs per day on average.

Fennel

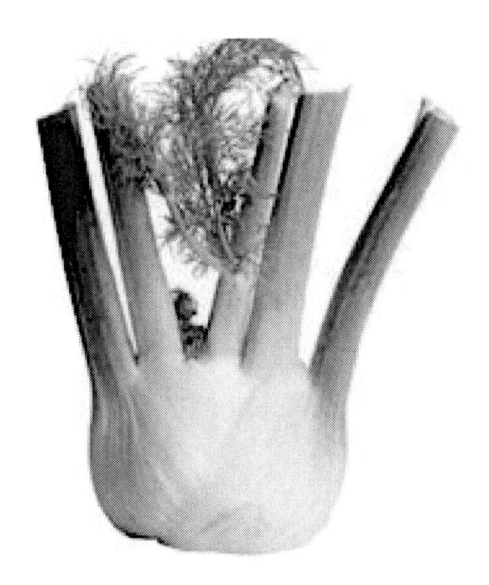

Fennel contains significant amount of vitamin C, and is also a source of fibre, potassium and folate. In addition, it contains a range of phytochemicals including anethole and other terpenoids which have shown a number of anti-cancer, anti-inflammatory and digestive benefits.

Anethole in particular, has been shown in studies to reduce a potentially harmful protein complex called NF-kappaB (NF-kB), which triggers genetic change and inflammation. This protein is persistently active in cases of cancer, arthritis, inflammation, asthma, neurodegenerative diseases and more.

Figs

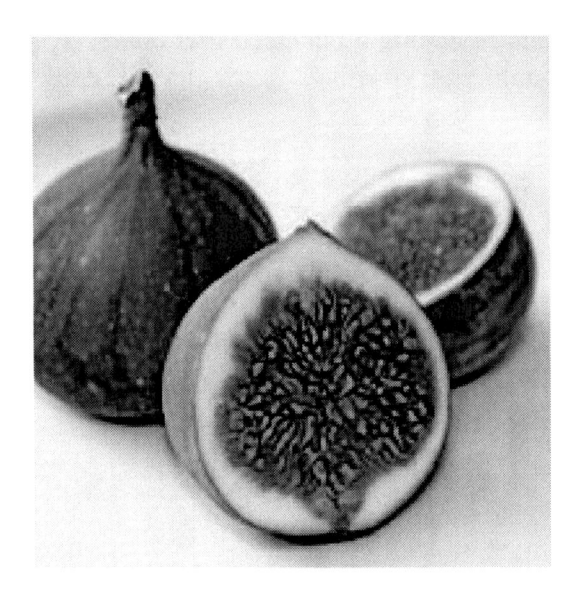

Figs have the greatest amount of fibre, in comparison with any other fresh or dried fruit, which makes them excellent for your digestive system. They also contain digestive enzymes that promote regular bowel movement. This helps to reduce the risk of colorectal cancer.

Figs also contain a number of antioxidants, which help to protect your cells and DNA from free radical damage.

Fish

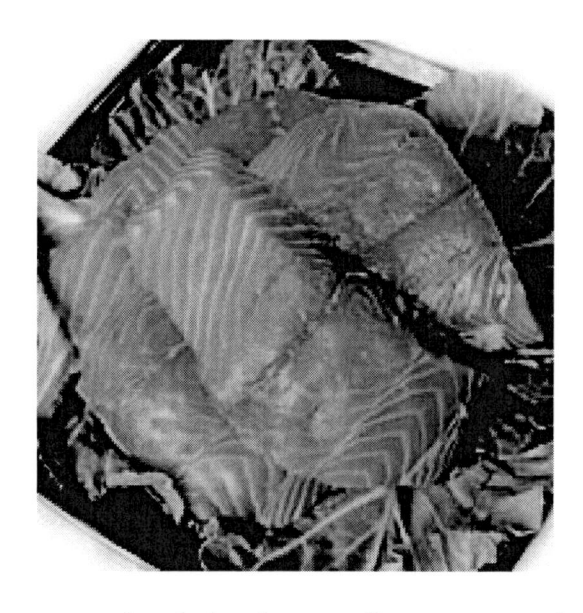

Wild salmon, mackerel, herring, sardines, tuna and any other kinds of oily fish are excellent sources of omega-3 and omega-6 fatty acids.

The brain contains high levels of omega-3 fat, so consistent ingestion of foods containing omega-3 fatty acids is vital for brain function. Deficiency can present itself in the form of low attention span, poor memory, learning difficulties and a reduction in heart health.

Omega-3 found in oily fish is converted into prostaglandins, which lubricate the eyes, arteries and your joints. It also strengthens the roots of your hair and makes your hair more shiny by encouraging natural oil production.

It is also thought to play a part in the function of your immune system. A study published in the journal "Paediatrics" on over 1000 pregnant women showed that mothers consuming daily supplementation of these essential fatty acids during pregnancy, gave birth to significantly healthier babies.

The babies at the age of one month, where 25% less likely to develop cold symptoms, and when they did, they had a shorter duration of coughs, phlegm, and wheezing.

At the age of three months, the group of babies whose mothers had been supplemented, were ill 14% less often.

The babies were also, the researchers noted, 100g heavier at birth on average, and almost a centimetre longer (taller) than average at the age of 18 months.

Oily fish are also some of the few places you can obtain vitamin D from your diet. Usually, you manufacture vitamin D in your skin through Sun exposure. However, if you do not get enough sun, you run the risk of having insufficient vitamin D. This is where adding fish to your diet can greatly increase your health - particularly in colder countries where sun exposure is reduced.

Insufficient vitamin D levels are linked to pretty much every age-related disorder there is, including heart disease, cancer, chronic inflammation, depression, autoimmune diseases, diabetes and osteoporosis. If you have to obtain your vitamin D from your diet, try to cook your fish with coconut oil, because polyunsaturated oils hinder the binding of vitamin D to D-binding proteins that allow the vitamin to be used in your body.

If you can't bring yourself to consume greater quantities of fish, then organic Flaxseed oil is a good supplement for the omega-3 and omega-6 essential fatty acids. Combine this with a supplement containing vitamin D3 (cholecalciferol) to obtain many of the benefits. Be aware however, that vitamin D2, a synthetic form of vitamin D is not the same and has not been shown to have the same anti-cancer benefits.

You should also bear in mind that not all fish are equal. For example, farmed salmon does not have the same health benefits as wild salmon. Many farmed fish contain dangerously high levels of mercury and other contaminants such as pesticides and antibiotics. A study carried out in the UK in 2001, discovered that farmed salmon could contain as much as 10 times more dioxins and PCBs than wild salmon (both of which are carcinogenic). These are waste products and pollution relating to the manufacturing of plastics, and the residues from insecticides.

The dangers of these particular compounds is that they cannot be broken down within the body, so they can build up to dangerous levels.

The best way to avoid this is to buy ocean caught fish, such as wild Alaskan salmon. The added advantage is that it can contain as much as three times greater levels of omega-3 oils, along with higher levels of antioxidants.

Flaxseed or Linseed

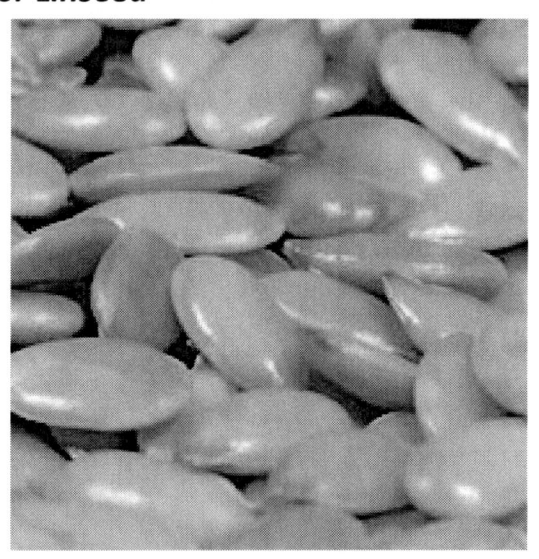

Flaxseed, otherwise known as Linseed, contains the same essential fatty acids as oily fish (but not the vitamin D3), so it can be a great supplement if you would rather get your essential fatty acids from a vegetarian source. Please see the Fish section for details on the effect of these essential fatty acids.

The fibre components of Flax, Lignans, have also demonstrated that they can slow tumour growth in prostate and breast cancer patients.

Studies on mice have shown that flaxseed can improve the effectiveness of the cancer drug tamoxifen. Scientists have also discovered that women with a high level of enterolactone (which is associated with a high lignan intake from foods such as flax), experienced a decrease in their breast cancer risk by 58%. Other sources of lignans and enterolactone include brown rice and rye.

An animal study discovered that supplementing flaxseed oil was effective in helping to prevent colon tumour development. Corn oil, on the other hand, which contains mostly omega-6 fatty acids actually promoted tumour growth.

In studies related to diabetes, adding Flax to the diet of animals, was shown to slow the onset of type II diabetes and protect kidneys from the usual damage caused by the onset of the disease.

Whilst flaxseed oil is available in gelatin capsules, the greatest health benefits are from ground flax seeds because it contains all of the fibre and other plant compounds. You can sprinkle ground flax seeds on cereal, salads, soups, casseroles and any other meals you prepare.

Garlic

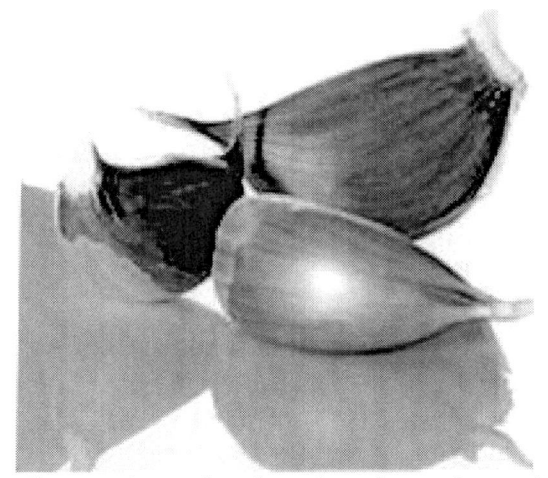

Although garlic may have developed a stigma due to its aroma, it is a food with a number of cancer-fighting compounds. Garlic contains selenium, which can block early stage breast cancer and contains organosulphur compounds that have many health benefits, including inhibiting cancer.

Well over 20 studies have shown that garlic has a range of anti-cancer effects, with particularly strong evidence for the prevention of prostate and stomach cancers.

A recent study involving over 1000 healthy female twins also uncovered the fact that women who consume diets high in garlic, leeks and onions (known as allium vegetables) have significantly lower levels of osteoarthritis in their hips, knees and spine. It is believed that this is due to a compound called diallyl disulphide which limits cartilage-damaging enzymes.

Garlic also has been shown in studies to boost immunity by stimulating natural killer cells, it reduces the risk of atherosclerosis, heart disease, stroke, colds and flu and has been found beneficial for those suffering from stroke, bronchitis, asthma, stomach ulcers, worms, and more.

One of the main ingredients that yields the greatest health benefits from eating garlic is a substance called allicin. However, allicin is not actually present in garlic. It comes from the alliin in garlic being mixed with an enzyme in garlic called allinase. This happens when the garlic is chewed, cut or bruised.

So if you want to be sure you get the benefits of garlic on a daily basis without actually eating it, you can consume a supplement, but be sure to use allicin powder extract, because garlic powder, garlic oil, and garlic tablets do not typically contain much stable and bioavailable allicin.

According to a study published in the Journal of Agricultural and Food Chemistry in 2001, when numerous brands of garlic supplement were tested, 83% of them yielded less than 15% of the potential allicin.

Garlic macerates contain a low level of allicin, but allicin powder extracts are much better - greater even than consuming garlic itself.

I use a supplement called Alliforce™ which is 100% allicin that has been stabilised for bioavailability and is not affected by stomach acid. With 270mg of allicin in each capsule, it has over 100 times more allicin than many other garlic supplements.

http://www.CancerUncensored.com/recommended-products

Ginger Root.

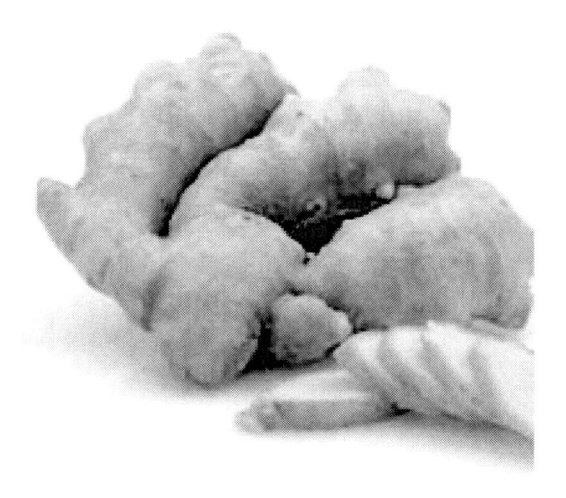

Ginger has long been known to possess a number of therapeutic properties. It is being used in remedies for coughs, colds, sore throats, bronchitis, and even to reduce nausea. However, a recent study published in Cancer Prevention Research, a journal of the American Association for Cancer Research, indicated that it also could be used as a supplement to prevent colon/bowel cancer.

Participants in the study were noted as having significantly reduced markers of colon inflammation. Such inflammation has been shown in prior studies to be a significant precursor to colorectal cancer.

The levels of Ginger Root used in the study were 2g of ginger extract, which is the equivalent to eating 20g of raw ginger.

Other US studies have also shown ginger to have powerful anti-inflammatory properties which can help to relieve the discomfort from arthritis, and more importantly where cancer is concerned, gingerols, an active ingredient within ginger, have been shown to kill cancer cells.

Interestingly, a US study indicated that ginger was just as effective in the treatment of arthritis as the standard and currently available anti-inflammatory drugs, but did not display any of the dangerous side effects.

In a study conducted by the University of Michigan, ginger was found to be excellent at killing cancer cells. When researchers dissolved ginger powder into a solution containing ovarian cancer cultures, the mutated cells died.

It was found that the ginger destroyed the ovarian cancer cells in two different ways. Firstly, the ginger triggered programmed cell death, (apoptosis), and secondly, the ginger triggered autophagy, which is where the cancer cells digest themselves. The researchers discovered that ginger caused the exact same rate of apoptosis that chemotherapy drugs achieve, yet ginger does not cause any side-effects. The researchers also highlighted the fact that Ginger Root helps to control inflammation, which can be a precursor to ovarian cancer.

Goji Berries

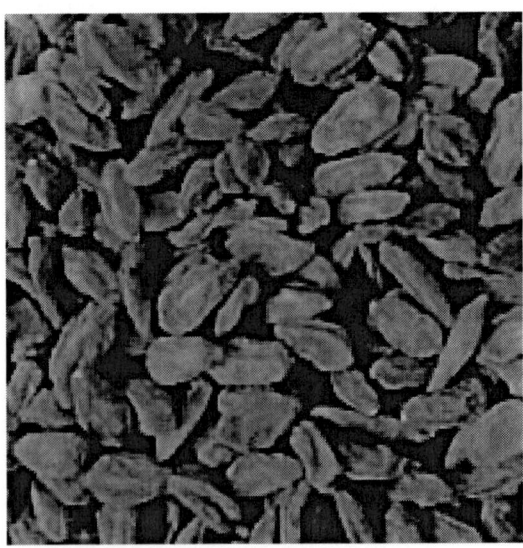

Goji berries are a little-known berry from Tibet and inner Mongolia. They are small and orangey red in colour, with a taste somewhere between cherry and cranberries. Typically they are dried, at which point they are similar in size to raisins.

Whilst they aren't rich in any one particular vitamin or mineral, they do contain high levels of beta carotene and zeaxanthin.

In studies, an extract of the Goji berry were shown to stop the spread of liver cancer cells, and triggered cancer cell death. Other studies have shown that Goji berries inhibited leukaemia cancer cells, and a further study, conducted on mice, demonstrated that Goji extract improved upon the cancer killing effect of radiation therapy.

In addition to purchasing the dried berries, they can be purchased as powder or juice. They are delicious when added to breakfast cereals, or even rice pudding, but I mix them in with other nuts and seeds to add variety.

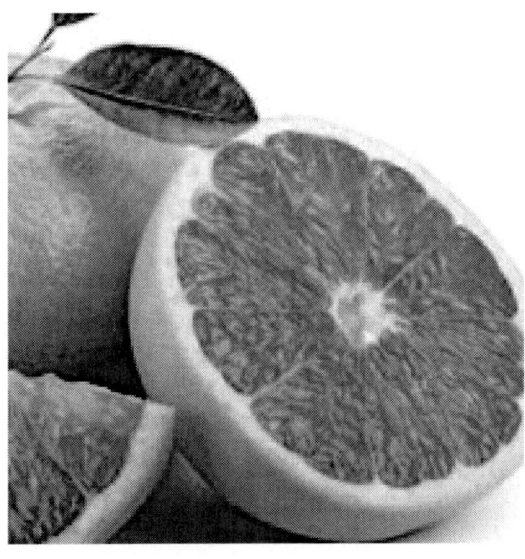

Grapefruit

Grapefruit are an excellent source of vitamin C, but the red or pink versions are far superior in terms of their concentration of carotenoids, which act as powerful antioxidants. In fact, they can contain as much as 50 times more than white grapefruit. In addition to the vitamin A, calcium, potassium and other nutrients, grapefruit contain more than 150 phytonutrients which have been shown to help with anti-ageing, cancer, ulcers, heart disease, allergies and fighting infections.

A study showed that one of the flavonoids found in grapefruit helps to repair damaged DNA in human prostate cancer cells. Researchers also found that including grapefruit in the diet of rats, reduced the inflammatory markers associated with colon cancer and increased programmed cell death.

In another study, conducted upon patients who had undergone heart bypass surgery, researchers discovered that eating a red grapefruit each day for 30 days reduced the patient's total cholesterol, LDL (bad) cholesterol and triglycerides, which would aid in their recovery.

In a study relating to weight loss, whereby overweight individuals ate half of a fresh grapefruit before meals for a period of 12 weeks, it was determined that they lost additional weight over the group who did not consume grapefruit. Using grapefruit as a fad diet, such as those developed in Hollywood, is not a good plan, but adding it to meals is likely to increase your health and weight loss results.

Just be aware that grapefruit juice can influence the rate at which you absorb certain medications, so please check with your doctor or pharmacist if grapefruit will interfere with any medication you are taking.

Grapes and grape juice

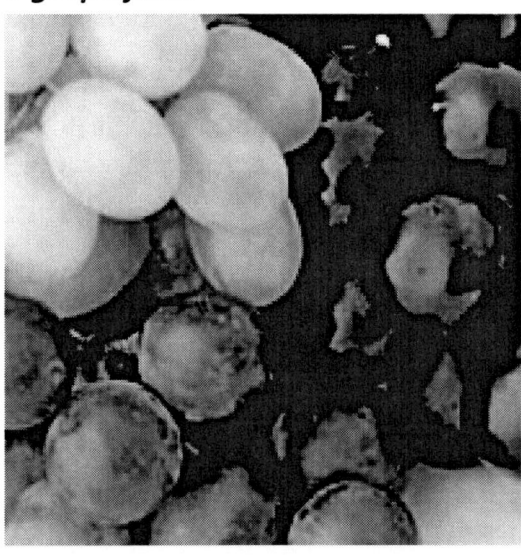

Grapes are a good source of flavonoids, vitamin C and potassium, with a modest amount of fibre. The skin of grapes contains a phytonutrient called resveratrol, which has been shown to have anti-inflammatory and cancer fighting properties. Red grapes also contain lycopene, which is a carotenoid you also find in tomatoes. Studies indicate that lycopene may help in fighting breast and prostate cancer.

Interestingly, grape seeds contain a large amount of very effective antioxidants. The most potent of these, proanthocyanidin, has 20 times more antioxidant power than vitamin E, and over 50 times more antioxidant power than vitamin C! On that basis, it makes sense to eat grapes complete with seeds, rather than opting for seedless varieties.

A variety of studies have shown that grapes are useful in cancer prevention, and that grapes or grape extracts can inhibit the growth of cancer cells including cancers of the breast, stomach, colon, prostate and leukaemia.

In a study conducted on human advanced prostate cancer cells, it was shown that grape seed extract not only inhibited cell growth, but also caused them to die.

A study on red wine discovered that individuals consuming four or more glasses of red wine each week reduced their risk of prostate cancer by 50%.

Where heart health is concerned, studies using freeze-dried grape powder demonstrated that LDL cholesterol could be prevented from converting to the more dangerous type that leads to heart disease, whilst simultaneously increasing the levels of good HDL cholesterol.

In a further study, it was discovered that grape juice significantly improved short-term memory of laboratory animals, along with improving their coordination, strength and balance.

Green Tea

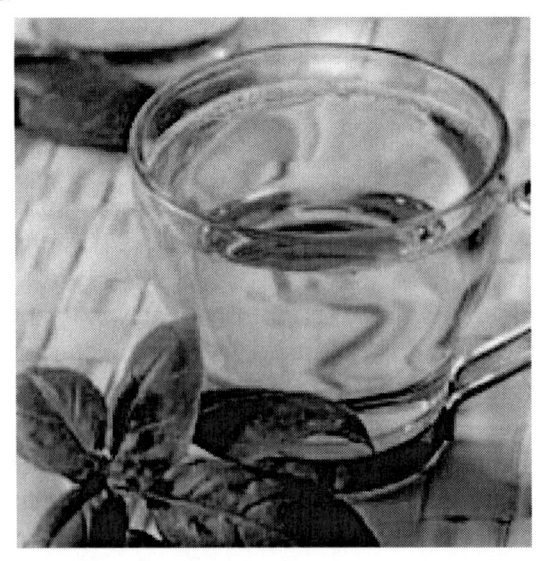

If you are a regular drinker of tea or coffee, try using decaffeinated green tea as a substitute. Green tea contains catechins such as EGCG, (Epigallocatechin gallate), as well as other anti-cancer bioflavinoids.

In a recent study, published in the journal Immunology Letters, 2011, they discovered that EGCG significantly increased the number of regulatory T cells, which are responsible for boosting immune system function, which is vital in your body's defence against cancer.

A 15 year study, which followed 61,057 women with ages ranging from 40 to 76, discovered some tremendous reductions in ovarian cancer risk when green tea was consumed regularly. They found that those women who consumed a cup of green tea every day, reduced their risk of ovarian cancer by 24%. Two or more cups per day, reduced the women's risk by 46%. Those study participants who consumed green tea consistently for a 30 year period, had an ovarian cancer risk reduction of 75%.

Not only do the powerful antioxidants limit the impact of free radicals, but they are also known to repair DNA damage. Other studies have shown that green tea can hinder the growth and spread of cancer cells by increasing programmed cell death, (apoptosis).

Whilst this major study concentrated primarily on ovarian cancer, other studies have shown that EGCG can help in the fight against other forms of cancer, including bladder, cervical, prostate and brain cancer. It also reduces inflammation and inhibits a protein, (Bcl-xl), that prevents programmed cell death in cancer cells.

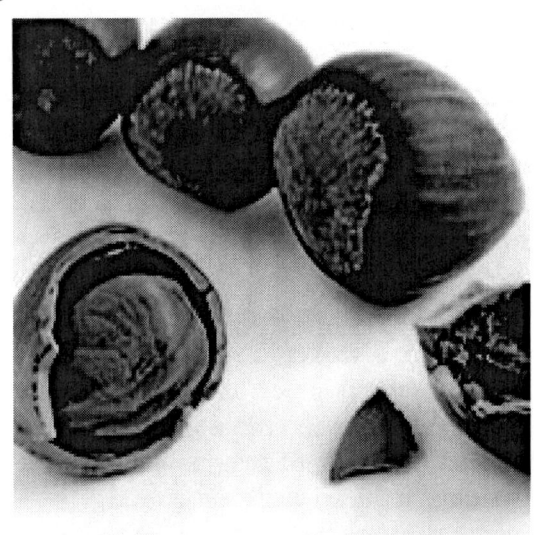

Hazelnuts

Hazelnuts contain substantial amounts of vitamin E, which is a powerful antioxidant. It also contains the largest concentration of folate amongst tree nuts. Folate is so important because it significantly reduces the risk of birth defects and has been linked, in a number of studies, to protecting against certain forms of cancer, depression, Alzheimer's disease and can boost heart health.

The minerals calcium, potassium, magnesium, and the amino acid arginine, are present within hazelnuts. They also contain proanthocyanidins, which are the same flavonoids contained in green tea that help to protect against allergy symptoms and improve circulation.

They are also high in protein and contain a substantial amount of fibre, which is necessary to protect against bowel cancer.

Studies have shown that hazelnuts can help reduce the risk of cataracts. One study in particular, (which I found rather distasteful), revealed that a group of rats were deliberately administered the chemotherapeutic drug doxorubicin in order to give them cataracts. Those rats that were consuming hazelnuts did not form cataracts like the other rats. The researchers theorised that the prevention of cataract formation was associated with the vitamin E and other phytochemicals found in hazelnuts.

According to the Journal of the National Cancer Institute, a government study of nearly 30,000 men showed that vitamin E supplements (taken at 400 IU per day), cut the prostate Cancer risk for smokers by 71%.

Another study published in the International Journal of Cancer in 2008, highlighted the significant differences in effectiveness of different kinds of vitamin E. There are four different kinds of Tocopherol (vitamin E) - alpha, beta, gamma and delta. The study found that increasing alpha-tocopherol consumption to 7.73mg per day or greater resulted in a 34 to 53% reduction in lung cancer risk. Beta, gamma and delta tocopherols did not have the same dramatic effect. So if you do supplement with vitamin E, make sure it is the alpha-tocopherol you are using. Other studies which have been used to refute the effectiveness of vitamin E, did not draw the distinction between the different forms.

Honey

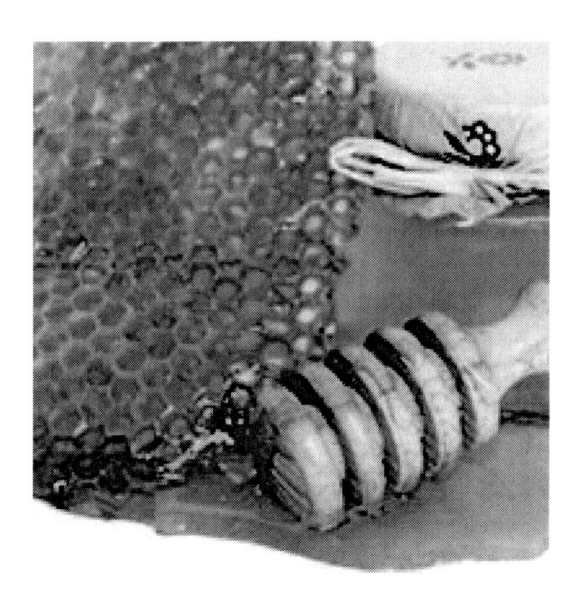

The benefits of honey have been discussed in the ancient texts of the Sumerians, Babylonians, Egyptians and more, because honey isn't just a natural sweetener.

Whilst it is primarily composed of fructose, glucose and water, honey also contains enzymes, minerals (including calcium, copper, manganese, magnesium, iron, phosphorus, zinc and potassium), vitamins, amino acids, flavonoids and phenolic acids. As a general rule of thumb, the darker the honey, the greater the level of antioxidants it contains. It also acts as a prebiotic, meaning that it aids in the growth and proliferation of friendly gut bacteria which help you to digest your food and boosts your immune system.

In the Journal of the Science of Food and Agriculture, it was reported that honey (administered orally and by injection) was effectively used to decrease tumour growth and suppress the spreading of cancer in mice.

Certain kinds of honey, especially Manuka honey (which comes from the Manuka Bush in New Zealand) have been found to be remarkably effective in treating infection and wounds, because it contains certain enzymes that are hostile to bacteria. Manuka Honey has been shown to even be able to kill MRSA, which is the antibiotic resistant bacteria associated with many hospital infections. A notable study conducted at Manchester hospital in the UK demonstrated that bandages soaked in Manuka Honey given to cancer patients after surgery, significantly reduced the incidence of MRSA infection and reduced inflammation.

A study conducted in 2003, published in the European Journal of Medical Research, which focused on post-operative infections (infected hysterectomy wounds and Caesarean section wounds), showed that where conventional treatments for wound infection only resulted in a 50% success rate, Manuka Honey resulted in an 85% success rate.

Manuka Honey is now licensed for use within National Health Service hospitals for dressing wounds. You can purchase it at different strengths, based upon what they call a "Unique Manuka Factor" rating, or UMF. The UMF rating is also sometimes referred to as the NPA rating or Non-Peroxide Activity rating.

Manuka Honey with a UMF5 (or NPA5) is equivalent to 5% standard antiseptic solution. Honey with a UMF rating of 10 is equivalent to 10% standard antiseptic solution, etc.

UMF10 and below are used for general digestive health, UMF15 is for diarrhoea, heartburn and indigestion. UMF20 can treat stomach ulcers or gastroenteritis.

Given the extraordinary benefits of a good quality honey, you should try to use honey as a sweetener instead of processed, refined white sugar (which has no other health benefits). As an extra bonus, you only need around half the amount.

Finally, consuming honey from your local area will help if you have allergies such as hay fever, because the pollen within it helps to desensitise you to your allergies.

However, please be aware that you should not give honey to infants less than a year old, because they are not yet able to kill the botulism spores that may be present.

Jalapeños

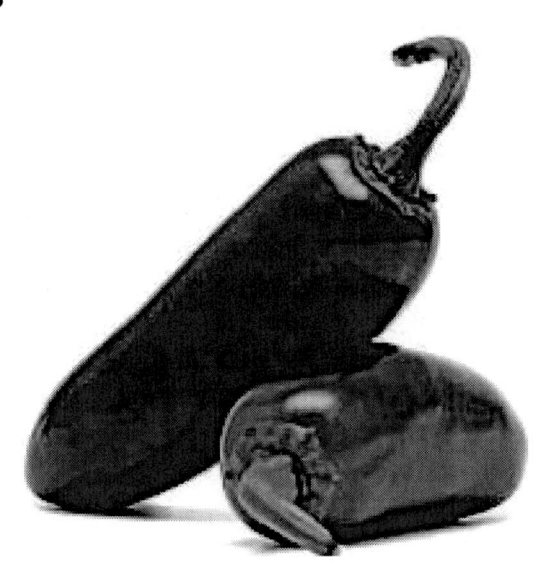

Jalapeño peppers contain vitamin C, vitamin A, and capsaicin, which is the component of peppers that gives you the "hot" sensation. Please see the Chilli Peppers section for more information on its positive effects on heart health, and cancer.

Kale

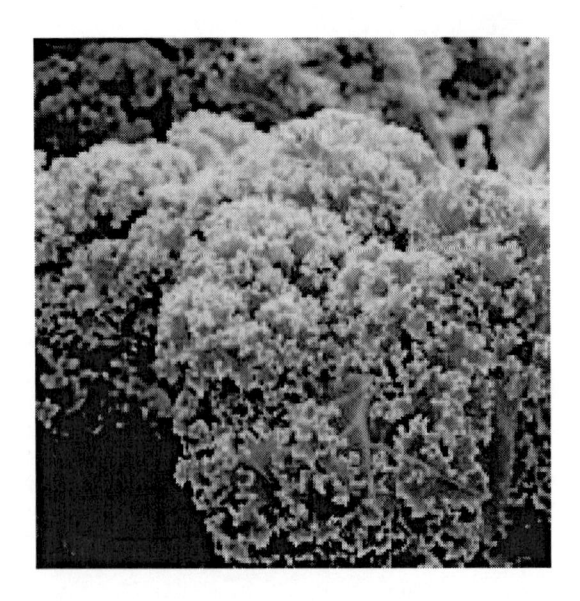

Kale is high in folate, which is vital in preventing blood vessel and DNA damage. It is a member of the cabbage family, so it also includes a number of the anti-cancer properties of broccoli, cauliflower, cabbage and brussels sprouts.

In addition to the folate, it is a good source of vitamin A, vitamin C, potassium, calcium, iron and a range of phytochemicals including lutein which promotes eyesight and has been shown to be beneficial in cancer studies.

According to the American Cancer Society, the carotenoids in Kale, have been shown to lower the risk of a range of cancers including mouth and pharynx cancers, oesophageal cancer and lung cancer. Other studies show similar properties with respect to bladder cancer.

Power combination: be sure to eat kale alongside foods rich in vitamin C, as this helps the absorption of the iron. Equally, adding oil, such as cold-pressed olive oil will help the absorption of the carotenoids.

Kidney Beans

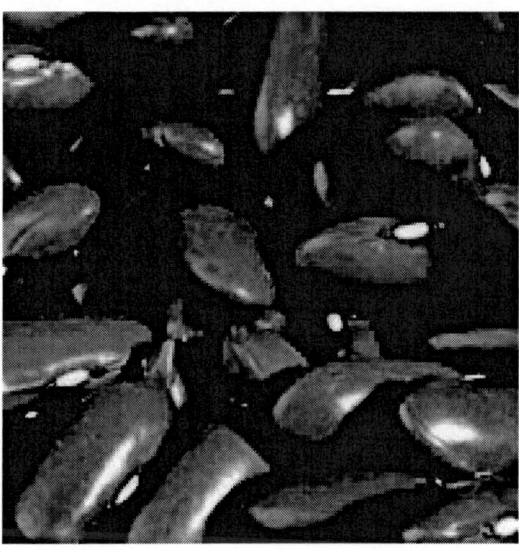

Kidney beans, chickpeas and lentils are all very rich in iron, which is essential for healthy red blood cells and energy levels. It is important to ensure that your iron levels are not depleted, because it will affect the oxygenation levels of your blood. Cancer cells prefer a low oxygen environment, and respond very poorly to higher levels of oxygen.

Kidney beans also have the advantage of being quite filling, so they are excellent for bulking out vegetarian meals.

Power Combination: combine kidney beans with a good source of vitamin C, such as broccoli or red peppers. Vitamin C can triple your body's ability to utilise the iron in your diet.

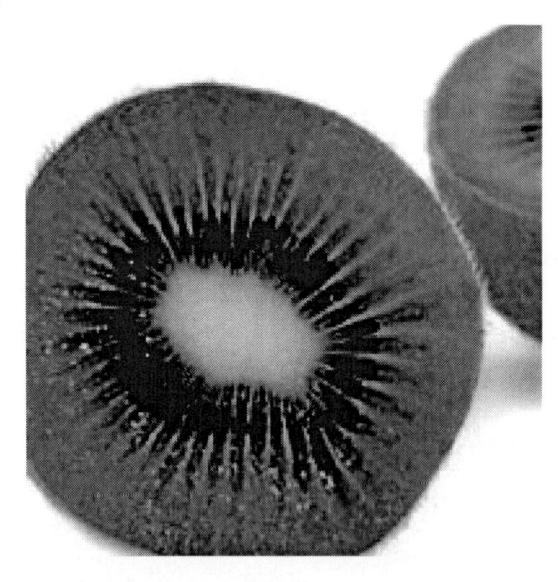

Kiwifruit

Kiwifruit has been quoted as being the most nutrient dense fruit out of 27 of the most commonly eaten fruits. It is particularly high in vitamin C, fibre, potassium and vitamin E. It also contains the phytochemical lutein, which may reduce the risk of cancer, heart disease and cataracts.

Like açai berries, blueberries and cherries, kiwifruit also contains anthocyanin, which is believed to provide protection against both cancer and heart disease.

Research at the Rowett Research Institute has shown that consuming kiwifruit as part of your daily diet can protect DNA from damage, and can actually help to repair existing DNA damage. Other studies have also shown that kiwifruit extracts can be effective in destroying oral tumour cells.

Recent studies on diets rich in lutein and zeaxanthin, have shown protective effects in relation to cataracts and other forms of macular degeneration, so Kiwis could be vital to maintaining your eyesight as you age. Add apricots as a source of vitamin A and carotenoids, and you have a serious combination to help your eyesight.

Lemons

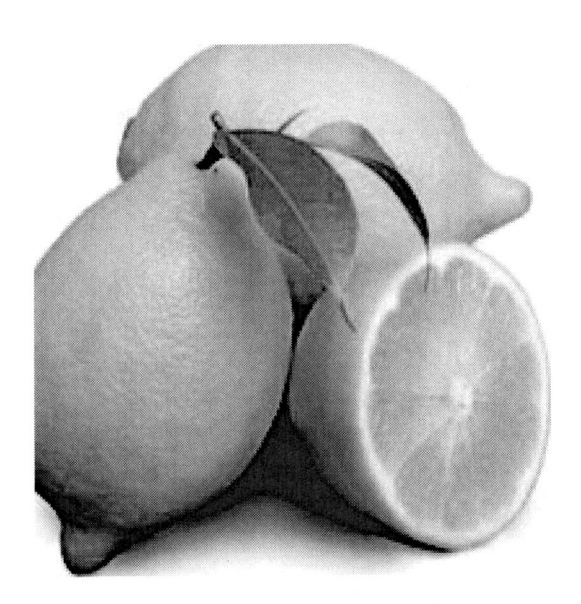

Lemons contain folate, vitamin C, vitamin A, potassium and a compound that has demonstrated anti-cancer properties called limonene. All citrus fruit are high in flavonoids, which are highly potent antioxidants.

In laboratory studies, citrus limonoids have been shown to exert an anti-proliferation effect on cancers of the colon, lung, breast, stomach, mouth, liver, skin and even human neuroblastoma tumours, which are more common in children.

Whilst cranberries were also shown to provide a benefit, lemons showed the greatest level of activity. It is believed that the difference in effectiveness is due to the fact that limonoids remain in the bloodstream for longer. Other products studied, such as the phenols in green tea, only remained in the bloodstream for 4 to 6 hours.

In relation to rheumatoid arthritis, a study involving over 20,000 people discovered that those who consumed the least foods rich in vitamin C were over three times more likely to develop arthritis than those who maintained a high vitamin C diet.

Add lemon to your drinks, squeeze fresh lemon juice over fish and salad and try to include lemon zest in your cookery.

Please also see the Citrus Fruit section for other fruit with similar properties.

Liquorice / Licorice

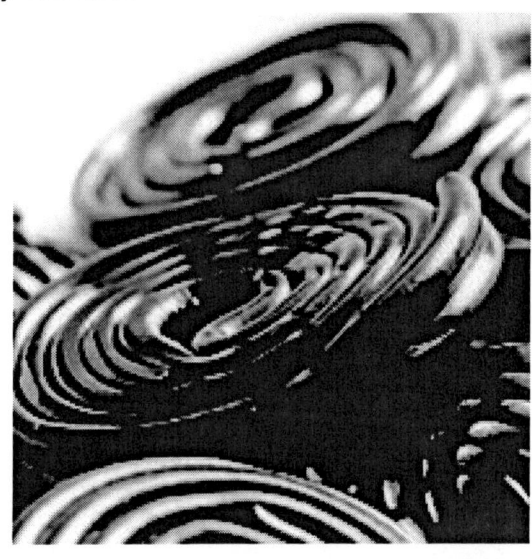

According to the American Cancer Society, "Laboratory studies have identified several substances in licorice that may help prevent DNA mutations, inhibit tumor formation, or even kill cancer cells. For example, Licochalcone-A, glabridin, and licocoumarone have been tested using cancer cells growing in laboratory dishes, and preliminary studies indicate that these chemicals can stop the growth of, or even kill, breast cancer, prostate cancer, and leukemia cells. In studies with mice, glycyrrhizin and glycyrrhizic acid reduced formation of skin, colon, liver, uterine, and breast cancers."

They went on to say "Although results of animal studies suggest some chemicals from licorice might be useful in preventing or treating some forms of cancer, no human clinical trials of licorice supplements or substances from licorice have been reported."

In a study published by the Journal of Clinical Investigation, scientists used glycyrrhizic acid, which is the main sweet-tasting component of liquorice, to block an enzyme that is critical for bowel cancer growth. The result was that the development of polyps was prevented in laboratory mice predisposed to bowel cancer, and the progression of bowel cancer was ceased.

While there may not be human clinical data available yet, treating yourself to some liquorice is likely to be beneficial.

Mangoes

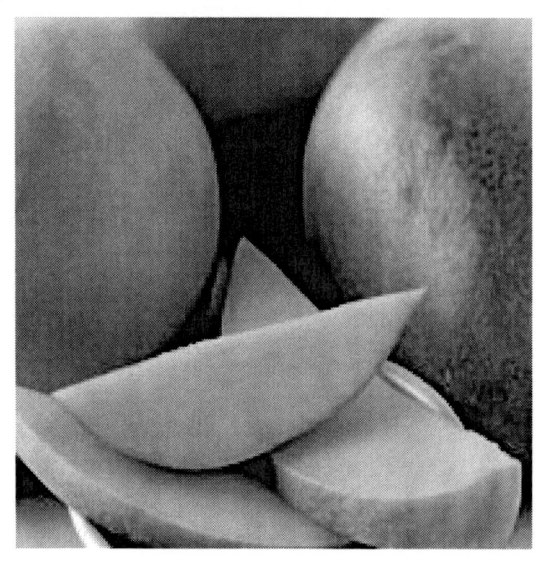

Mangoes are rich in vitamin A, vitamin C and beta-carotene, so if you aren't getting enough carrots, peppers or sweet potatoes, this is a viable alternative. In cancer cell studies, mangoes have been found to interrupt a number of different phases of growth throughout the life-cycle of cancer cells.

Mint

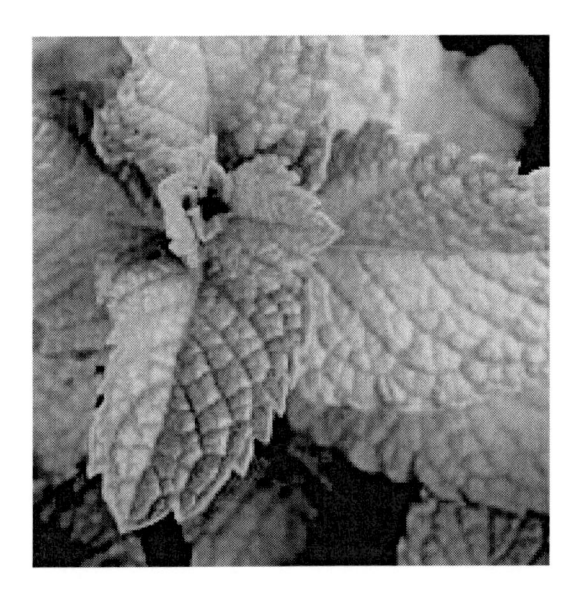

In addition to the numerous vitamins and minerals contained in mint, (including calcium, potassium, phosphorus, folate and vitamin A), the mint plant contains phenolic phytochemicals that act as antioxidants.

These phenolic compounds, along with high levels of salicylic acid, have shown in studies that mint can play a preventative role for both colorectal cancer and atherosclerosis. In other animal studies, a diet including mint was shown to significantly reduce the presence of lung cancer tumours in mice.

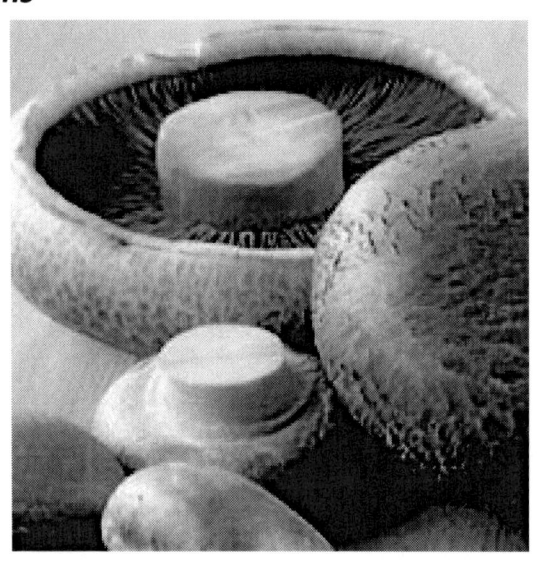

Mushrooms

Mushrooms aren't often thought of as being nutritionally dense, but in actual fact they are better than many other forms of fruit and vegetables for certain nutrients. They are a good source of B vitamins such as riboflavin, pantothenic acid, and some varieties of mushroom (including Portobello, Crimini and White mushrooms) are high in the mineral potassium.

Where cancer is concerned, the punch that mushrooms pack is in the form of vitamin D, various antioxidant polyphenols, and an antioxidant well-known for its anti-cancer properties called ergothioneine. Mushrooms are the only vegetarian source of high levels of vitamin D, with white button mushrooms being particularly high in it.

In a recent study published in the British Journal of Cancer, extracts from the mushroom Phellinus linteus were shown to halt the growth of breast cancer cells. Researchers theorised that the mushroom might stop an enzyme called AKT, (which is responsible for the development of new blood vessels within the tumour), from functioning properly.

This form of mushroom, (Japanese "meshimakobu", Chinese "song gen", Korean "sanghwang") is a medicinal mushroom that has been used in Japan, Korea and China for centuries. Nine different active compounds have been identified within it, but scientists are still researching which are responsible for stimulating the hormonal and cell-mediated immune function, which quenches inflammatory reactions, and which suppresses tumor growth and metastasis (spreading).

Another study, which tested seven different vegetable extracts, discovered that white mushroom extract was the most effective in inhibiting an enzyme associated with breast cancer growth called aromatase.

Along with these various cancer inhibiting chemicals, mushrooms also contain betaglucans and other substances that assist your immune system in recognising and eliminating abnormal cells.

White button mushrooms have also been shown to suppress the growth of androgen-independent prostate cancer cells and were responsible for a decrease in tumour size. The researchers suggested that white button mushrooms should be used as a dietary component to aid in the prevention of prostate cancer in men.

Nuts and seeds

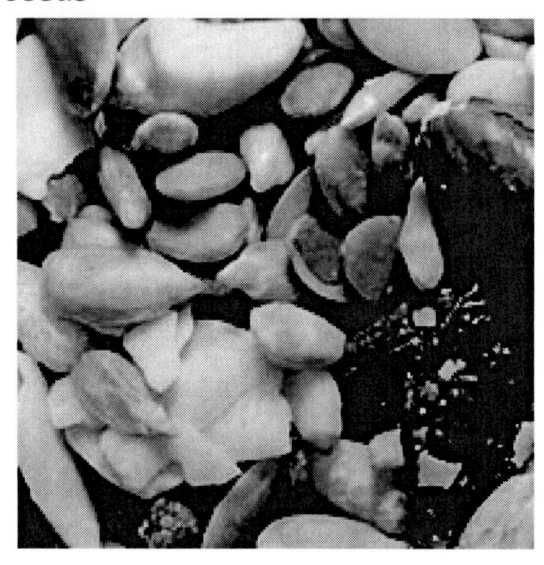

Please see Almonds, Brazil Nuts, Cashew Nuts, Hazelnuts, Walnuts, Pistachio Nuts, Sunflower Seeds, Pumpkin Seeds.

Olive oil

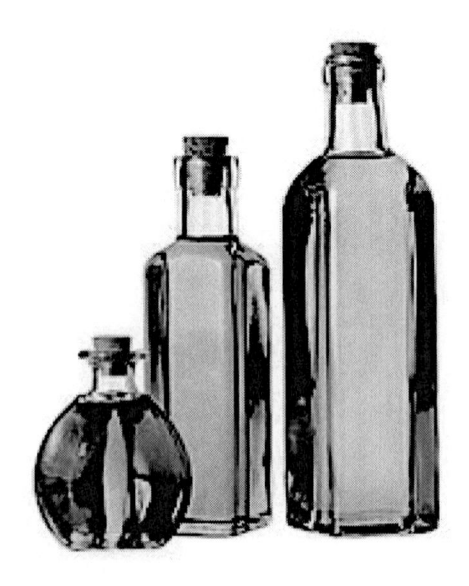

Research shows that olive oil can help to stunt the growth of tumours, and protects against damage to your DNA.

Previous studies have linked an olive oil-rich diet to a reduction in the likelihood of various different cancers forming, but only recently have they been able to theorise the reason for this.

In experimentation on rats, researchers were able to demonstrate that the olive oil influenced a gene that drives the growth of tumours; in this particular case, breast tumours. The gene switched off proteins that the cells were reliant upon for survival.

Olive oil is rich in vitamin E and other natural antioxidants. It also contains a compound called oleocanthal, which has significant anti-inflammatory properties. So not only does olive oil help in the fight against cancer, it also helps to reduce your risk of heart disease by lowering blood pressure.

Use cold-pressed olive oil for cooking at medium temperatures, and use cold-pressed extra virgin olive oil for salads, etc. Olive oil isn't suitable for high temperature cooking - in those cases, opt for cold-pressed coconut oil or cold-pressed rape seed oil, which have a much higher burning point. If oils are not cold-pressed, they have been heat treated, and this may make them harmful according to research by Dr Budwig.

Onions

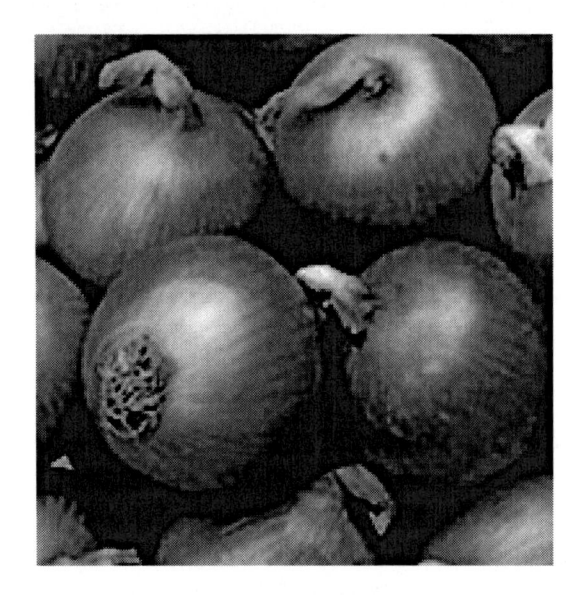

In addition to vitamin C and folate, onions are an excellent source of fibre. Even more importantly, where cancer is concerned, onions also contain allyl sulphides and flavonoids, such as quercetin, both of which are thought to reduce the risk of certain cancers.

In a study of 582 subjects, it was found that those people who increased their onion consumption, also decreased their risk of developing cancer. Another study, involving men from Finland, showed that those men who ate foods high in quercetin, (such as onions, apples, apricots, barley and cherries) reduced the incidence of lung cancer by 60%.

Researchers at Cornell University discovered that you get a greater level of inhibition of cancer growth (of liver and colon cancer cells) from stronger tasting onions than milder versions. New York bold, Western yellow and shallots were therefore more effective than other forms of onion.

Interestingly, allyl sulphides found in onions, also have been found to significantly lower LDL cholesterol levels, decrease the tendency to form blood clots, reduce atherosclerosis and reduce the risk of cardiovascular disease, stroke and heart attack. Add to that the fact that in rats, regular consumption of onion increases bone density and reduces the likelihood of osteoporosis, and you have a solid addition to a healthy diet.

Try to opt for red onions, as they also include the powerful antioxidant lycopene, which you also find in red peppers, tomatoes and other red fruit and vegetables.

Oranges

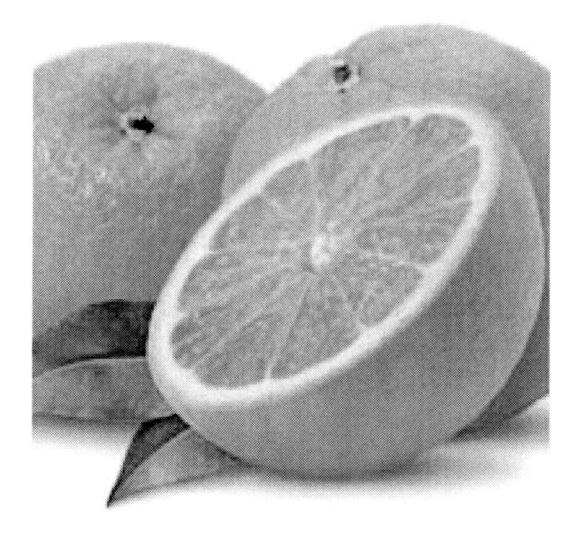

Oranges contain potassium, folate, vitamin C and are a rich source of flavanones, which act as antioxidants.

Studies have shown those people who consume oranges have elevated levels of citrate in their urine, which helps prevent kidney stones from forming.

The white fibres surrounding an orange also help to curb appetite and can suppress hunger levels for several hours after consuming them. Studies have indicated that those people who ate fresh fruit, including oranges, tended to eat less at subsequent meals, compared with those who ate junk food including crisps, crackers, candy or cakes.

Papayas

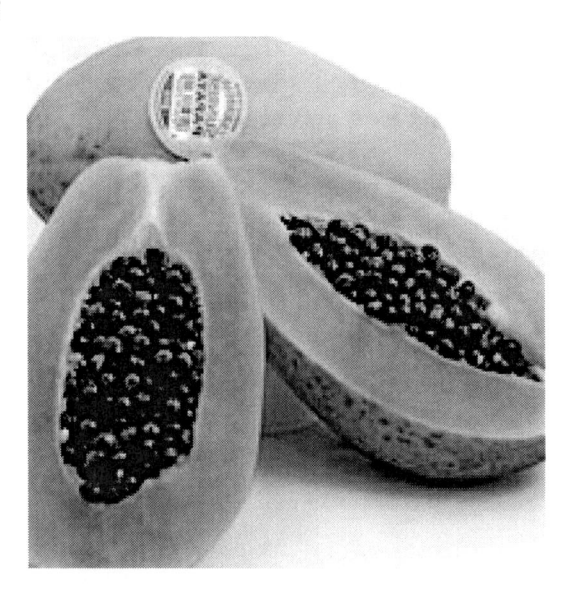

Papayas are a fruit which is less common to the Western diet than many others, however papayas contain a wide variety of nutrients, making this a worthy addition to your diet.

Papayas contain more vitamin C than oranges, and are good source of folate, fibre, vitamin A and potassium, along with various carotenoids including cryptoxanthin. Cryptoxanthin has been shown to reduce the risk of both colon and lung cancer, and may be beneficial for people with rheumatoid arthritis.

Interestingly, papaya also contains papain, a digestive enzyme that helps you break down protein. If you do not supplement with enzymes, consuming papaya with a meal will help you digest the meat component more effectively, improving bowel health.

A study, researching one of the primary causes of cervical cancer, the human papillomavirus (HPV), discovered an interesting link.

Women who were consuming elevated levels of beta-cryptoxanthin, vitamin C and lutein (all of which are present in papaya) had a lower risk of contracting the HPV virus that those who didn't. Just one papaya per week was enough to reduce a woman's risk of infection. By avoiding the HPV virus, this directly reduces the incidence of cervical cancer.

The aforementioned compounds also help to maintain better eyesight for longer, and may help reverse macular degeneration in older people.

Parsley

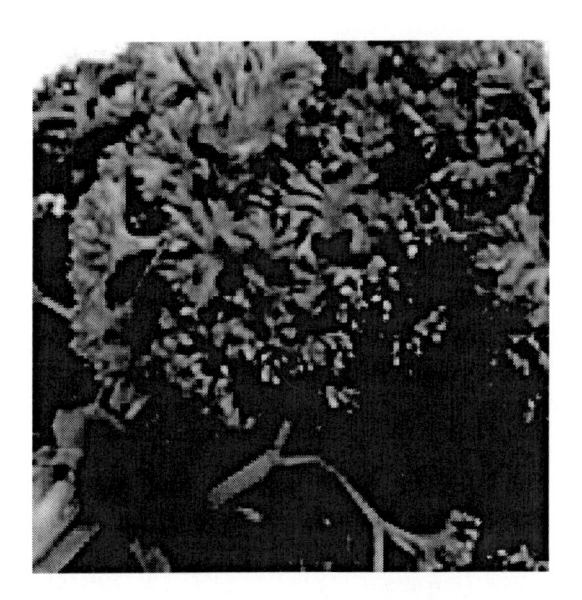

Belonging to the same family as both celery and carrots, parsley is usually found on the side of your plate as a garnish. However, you should actively try to include it in your diet.

Not only does it contain vitamin C, iron, iodine (which you also get in seaweed), and a range of other minerals, it also contains a range of phytochemicals with anti-cancer properties.

One in particular, myristicin, has been shown in mouse studies to be an effective inhibitor of tumours.

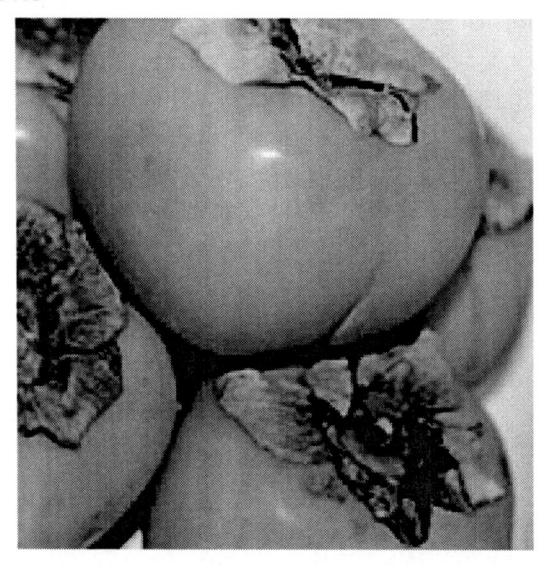

Persimmons

Persimmons, otherwise known as "kaki" or "Sharon fruit", are a great source of vitamin A and they also contain fibre, vitamin C and a range of phytochemical antioxidants. These antioxidants include gallic, epicatechin, proanthocyanidin and p-coumaric acids.

Two different studies have shown that persimmon extract strongly inhibited the growth of leukaemia cells, whilst also triggering apoptosis (programmed cell death).

Pistachio Nuts

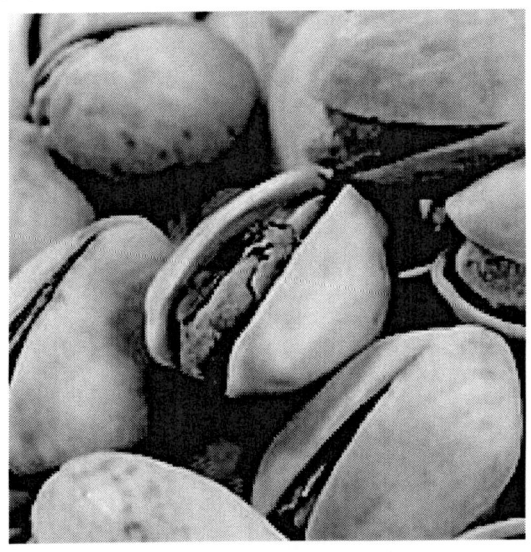

Of all of the tree nuts, pistachio nuts contain the highest levels of phytosterols, which have anti-cancer properties. They also contain the mineral calcium, which is anti-viral, as well as magnesium which helps you to absorb the calcium.

Magnesium also assists with reducing allergic reactions (which would otherwise hinder your immune system's ability to deal with cancer).

Added to that, the high levels of the amino acid arginine help your blood vessels to dilate, improving circulation and heart health. Pistachios also contain lutein, which is excellent for the health of your eyes.

Pomegranates

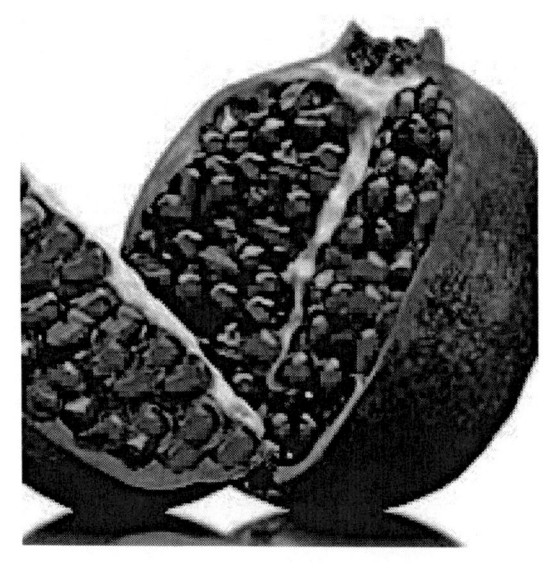

Pomegranates contain phytochemicals that have been shown to reduce the occurrence of hormone-dependent breast cancers. In particular, compounds known as ellagitannins, which suppress oestrogen production, help to stop the growth and spread of breast cancer cells and tumours, according to the results of a recent study.

Scientists have been aware of pomegranate's high antioxidant activity, which they believe is related to the high polyphenol content of the fruit, but it is only more recently that they have discovered that the polyphenol ellagic acid inhibits the enzyme aromatase which plays a key role in the development of breast cancer.

Pomegranates are also a rich source of vitamin B5, potassium and vitamin C. The seeds are also a great source of fibre.

Potatoes

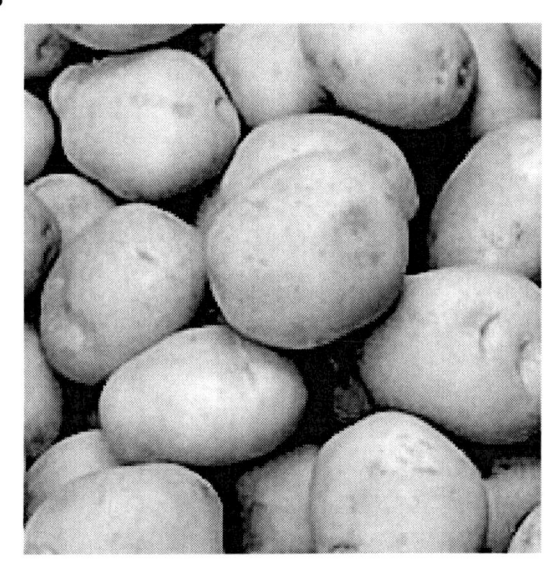

Potato has become a staple of Western diets, but people do not often consider the nutritional values of this vegetable. It is a far healthier alternative to Pasta or bread, because it contains vitamin C, potassium, fibre (in the skin) and antioxidants including anthocyanins and carotenoids - particularly in coloured potatoes.

Potatoes also contain lectins, which have been found, in human studies, to bind to the receptors on cancer cell membranes, leading to an inhibition of tumour growth and apoptosis (programmed cell death).

Potatoes have even been proven to reduce the plasma glucose in diabetic rats, drastically reducing frequent urination.

Probiotics and Prebiotics

Probiotics are the helpful bacteria that live in our gut. They help us to break down the food we eat, enabling us to maximise the nutritional value. They also compete with, and inhibit, any bad bacteria, which keeps us healthy, giving our immune system a boost.

These good bacteria have been responsible for improving our digestive health, skin conditions, inflammation, obesity and more. They also stimulate our bowels to produce more of the proteins that protect the mucous membranes. It is estimated that as much as 70% of our immune system is found in the gut. This translates to as much as three whole pounds of helpful bacteria in the average adult!

Unfortunately, the consumption of alcohol, antibiotics, irritable bowel disease, stress and weight loss can all reduce the number of these helpful bacteria, allowing harmful bacteria to multiply. In order to keep a healthy balance, you should consume probiotic supplements such as capsules containing Lactobacillus acidophilus. These can be found in any good health food store, or by visiting www.CancerUncensored.com

Certain strains of Lactobacillus acidophilus can naturally inhibit over 27 different kinds of pathogenic bacteria, including salmonella, E. coli, Shigella, along with inhibiting Candida albicans, making your gut a much healthier place.

Other sources of probiotics include live yoghurt cultures and some cheeses, but it is hard to determine what dose of viable bacteria you are getting from them.

Prebiotics are the non-digestible sources of food that the good bacteria thrive upon. Whilst these can be beneficial, I would always simply go straight to the source and consume a capsule a day that contains anywhere from 2 billion to 5 billion viable Lactobacillus acidophilus bacteria.

Prunes

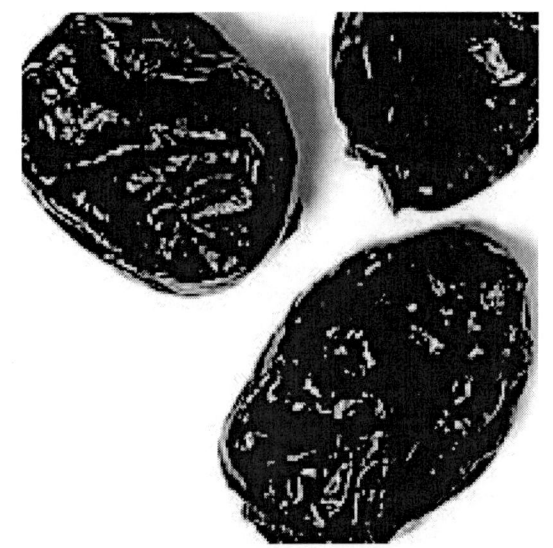

Prunes are dried plums. They contain very high levels of antioxidants. According to research carried out by the Human National Research Centre on Ageing at Tufts University, prunes were claimed to be excellent protection against premature skin ageing because they mopped up more free radicals (which damage your cells and tissues) than any other fruit they tested. They contain high levels of vitamin A, vitamin B6, iron and fibre to help maintain bowel regularity.

Regular bowel movements are very important to help reduce your risk of colorectal cancer.

Pumpkin and pumpkin seeds

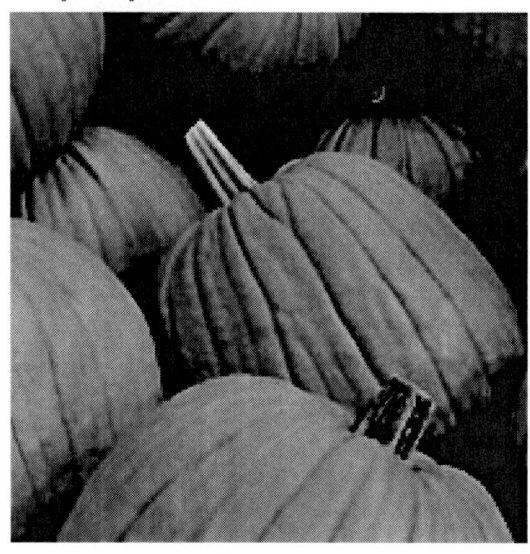

Pumpkins contain a wide variety of nutrients, including selenium, vitamin A, beta-carotene, beta-cryptoxanthin, lutein, potassium and fibre. The seeds of the pumpkin are also an excellent source of omega-3 fatty acids and phytosterols.

In Japan, a long-term study was conducted on 1352 colorectal cancer patients, 2455 breast cancer patients, 1398 lung cancer patients, 1988 gastric cancer patients, along with over 50,000 non-cancer outpatients. The study concluded that frequent consumption of pumpkin was linked to a decrease in risk across all four kinds of cancer.

A separate study also found a relationship between the consumption of pumpkin on a regular basis and a reduced risk of developing prostate cancer.

Power Combination: combine pumpkin seeds with butternut squash or other foods rich in beta-carotene such as sweet potato, carrot, spinach, mango and many of the other red, orange and green fruits and vegetables. Beta-carotene is converted into vitamin A, which is vital for healthy immune function. However, vitamin A will not work effectively without zinc, which is found in protein-based foods including pumpkin seeds.

Raspberries

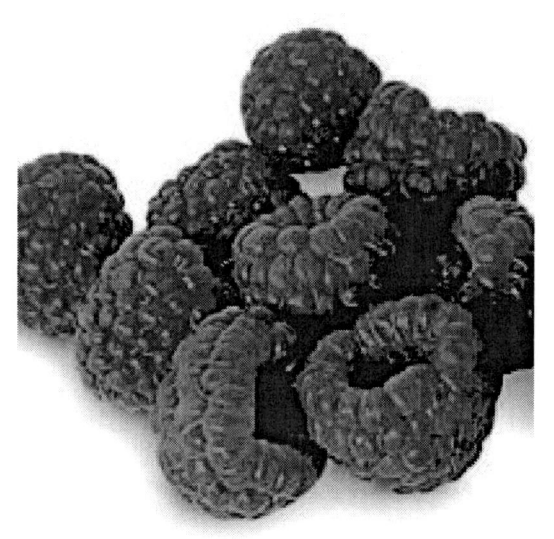

There are actually a wide variety of different raspberries, but many people are more familiar with the red variety, than the less common black raspberries found in North America.

Black raspberries can easily be confused with blackberries, but they are different. Blackberries are more shiny, and when you pick the fruit from the stem, black raspberries are hollow, whereas blackberries retain a central core from the plant.

Raspberries contain a generous amount of vitamin C, along with other nutrients such as selenium, phosphorus and dietary fibre. They are packed with antioxidants and a wide range of phytochemicals that are known to help prevent disease.

Freezing, drying or turning raspberries into preserves will reduce a significant proportion of the vitamin C, however the bulk of the antioxidants remain unharmed.

A number of studies have been conducted on raspberries, with particular attention paid to black raspberries, which have greater quantities of cancer-fighting substances.

One particular study, observing the effect of raspberry extracts on human liver cancer cells discovered that the more raspberry extract used, the less frequently the cancer cells replicated.

A study on human oesophageal cancer cells discovered that a diet containing black raspberries substantially reduced tumour cell growth.

Hamster studies have shown that black raspberries inhibit the formation of oral tumours.

Certain attention has been paid to the phytochemicals beta-sitosterol and ferulic acid (contained within black raspberries), because in studies it stopped the growth of both premalignant and malignant oral cancer cells.

In the field of diabetes, it has also been discovered that the anthocyanins in raspberries help reduce blood glucose levels after carbohydrate-rich meals. This will help to reduce the damage caused by excess levels of glucose, which causes the ageing of your tissues.

Laboratory studies using mice that were fed high-fat diets with varying quantities of raspberries discovered that greater raspberry consumption helps to prevent fatty livers and actually reduced the level of obesity.

Whilst your current consumption of raspberries may be limited to those contained in fruit yoghurt or preserves, you can purchase freeze-dried or frozen raspberries to add to your favourite desserts, or just to eat as a tasty treat.

Red grapes, red wine and grape juice

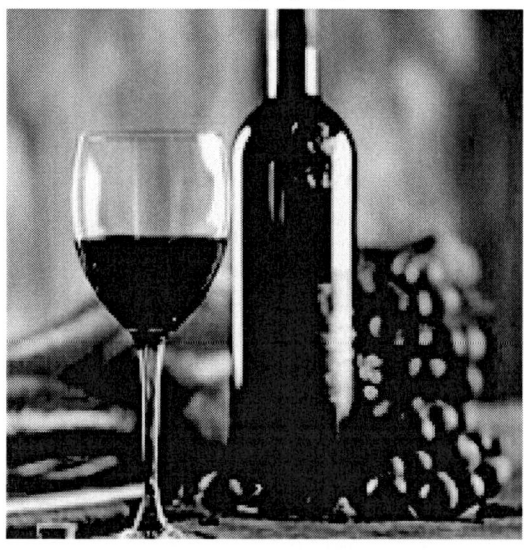

Grape skins contain resveratrol, a phytoalexin, and other potent anti-cancer chemicals. Grape seeds contain pycnogenol, which is reputed to have anti-cancer properties, so if possible, chew them rather than spitting them out.

Please see the Grapes section for more detailed information.

Rice (Brown Rice)

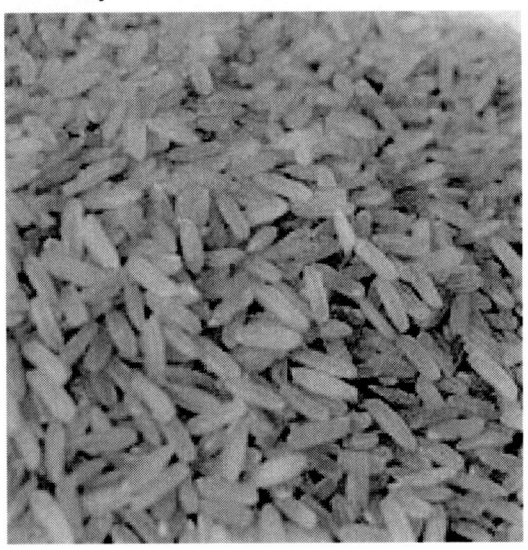

If you are choosing a source of carbohydrate to go with your meals, brown rice is an excellent choice over wheat-based products, such as pasta. Another great choice is sweet potato.

Brown Rice uses the whole grain, which contains numerous benefits related to heart health. In addition to the vitamin E, potassium, iron, phosphorus, thiamine, riboflavin and niacin, brown rice contains a range of lignans, phenolic compounds and phytoestrogens.

Just like flaxseed, brown rice contains lignans, including enterolactone, which helps your body establish the right kinds of healthy bacteria in your intestines, (which are credited with defending against a range of hormone-dependent cancers, including breast cancer).

A Danish study of postmenopausal women discovered that those women consuming the largest quantities of whole grains, including brown rice, were found to have significantly higher levels of enterolactone.

Previous studies have shown that women with a high level of enterolactone (which is associated with a high lignan intake from foods such as brown rice, flax and rye), experienced a decrease in their breast cancer risk by 58%.

Rosemary

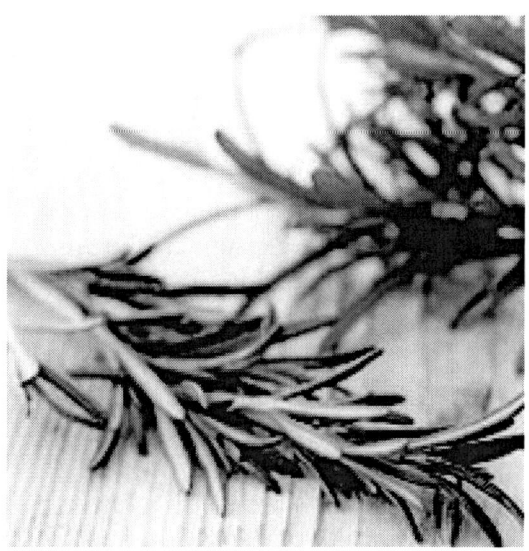

Rosemary is a herb native to the Mediterranean area. Belonging to the mint family, it contains a wide variety of polyphenolic compounds which act as antioxidants and have been shown to inhibit both bacterial growth and oxidation.

Rosemary is certainly something you should add to your diet, because in studies, it has shown a range of remarkable effects.

Extract of rosemary has been demonstrated to have a protective effect on human blood when it is exposed to gamma radiation. Other studies indicate strong anti-mutagenic properties, which enables your cells to resist genetic change and therefore prevent certain types of cancer.

One of the main polyphenol antioxidants in rosemary is carnosic acid. Cell studies show that when combined with vitamin D, carnosic acid reduces the spread of leukaemia cancer cells. This research is also being reinforced with the results from animal studies.

In studies conducted on mice fed a diet containing rosemary extract for 15 weeks, it was discovered that the number and size of their papillomas was reduced in comparison with control groups.

Rosemary may even be useful in protecting your lungs from environmental exposure to certain chemicals. In laboratory studies, mice were pretreated with an extract of Rosemary before being exposed to diesel exhaust fumes. The study discovered that those mice who had consumed the rosemary showed significantly less lung inflammation than the other mice.

Rosemary oil has been found to be particularly effective against E. coli bacteria, and may therefore also help to prevent bacterial growth in foods.

Whilst rosemary is available as fresh rosemary, dried, or as rosemary oil, I would always recommend fresh rosemary so that it retains both its flavour and its enzyme and phytochemical content.

Rye

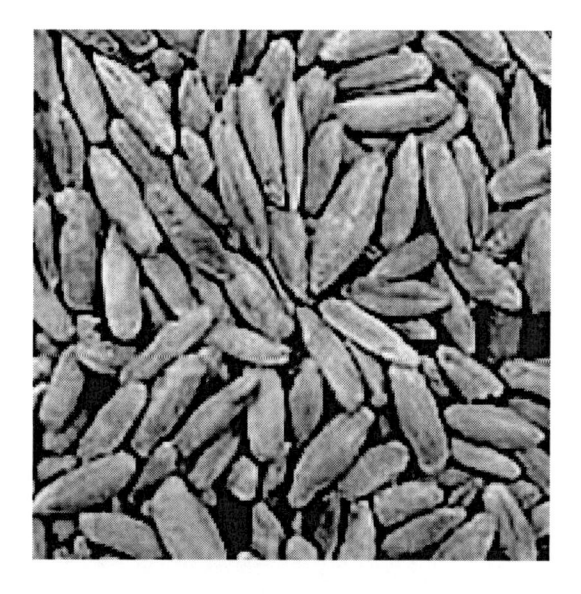

Rye is a form of cereal grain that is related to barley and wheat. It can be purchased as a whole grain, cracked, flour, flakes or already made into products such as rye bread.

Containing a number of important vitamins and minerals, including B vitamins, vitamin E, iron, zinc, folate, calcium, phosphorus, potassium and magnesium, rye also has a large concentration of lignans.

Just like flaxseed and brown rice, rye has shown significant digestive health benefits. In fact, one recent study indicated that fibre from rye appears to be more effective than whole grains from wheat in terms of the overall improvement of bowel health.

A study from Finland, researching serum levels of enterolactone, discovered that high levels of rye products correlated with high levels of enterolactone, which in turn correlated with a significant reduction in the risk of breast cancer.

Cell studies have shown that phytoestrogen and lignan extracts from rye, substantially inhibited the proliferation of cancer cells. In animal studies, rye bran was fed to mice that had developed prostate cancer. Researchers found that programmed cell death (apoptosis) within the tumours increased by over 30%, reducing tumour size by over 20%.

In a study focused on colon cancer, scientists found that by feeding mice a rye bran supplement for 12 to 31 weeks, they were able to significantly decrease the number of tumours found in the mice.

Seaweed

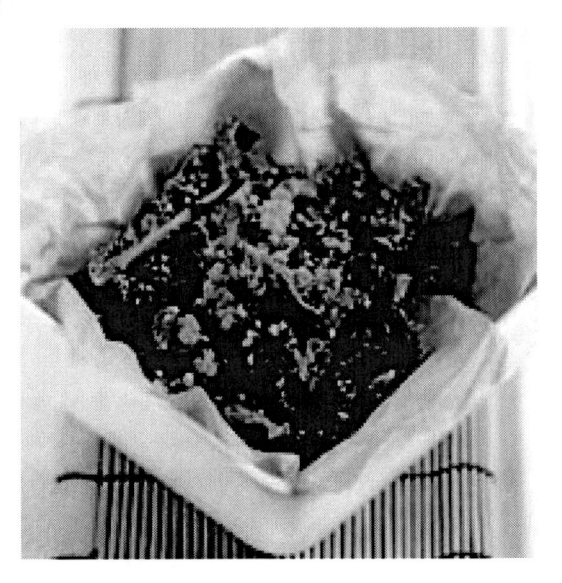

In the interests of simplicity, this section refers to edible seaweed or algae or any other ocean vegetables. These include kelp (wakame, arame, kombu), nori, dulse and sea lettuce (Monostroma and Ulva lactuca).

Seaweed is nutrient dense and is a source of a range of minerals including iodine, iron, calcium, and potassium. It can also be a good source of fibre.

In terms of vitamins and other micronutrients, different seaweed species contain varying amounts of vitamin C, vitamin A, vitamin B12, vitamin E, vitamin K, copper, zinc, selenium, manganese, magnesium and more. Brown seaweeds (such as wakame), have been shown to contain stearidonic acid, beta-carotene, fucoxanthin and violaxanthin, giving it antioxidant, anticoagulant, antibiotic and anti-inflammatory properties.

Brown seaweeds also contain Fucoidan, laminarin and alginic acid, which all exhibit anti-cancer properties in laboratory studies. The same can be said for the phlorotannins in kelp and phenolic acid in dulse.

Fucoidan, a polysaccharide found within brown seaweed, can make up to 4% of its total dry mass and this has been found to be a treasure trove for researchers. Numerous studies have been carried out, conclusively showing that this substance helps to modulate the immune system, support the health of normal cells, supports blood circulation, reduces cholesterol levels, improves joint mobility and stimulates immune response. On top of that, Japanese cell studies have shown that Fucoidan causes various different types of cancer to self-destruct, including certain kinds of leukaemia cells, colon cancer cells, stomach cancer cells and breast cancer cells.

Fucoidan has also been shown to be effective against lymphoma, whilst leaving healthy cells intact, in laboratory studies.

Brown seaweed, particularly wakame, also contains omega-3 fats including stearidonic acid and eicosapentaenoic acid which helps to balance out your omega-3 to omega-6 acid ratio. As per the section on Fish and Flaxseed, studies have shown that a high ratio of omega-6 to omega-3 in your diet can potentially increase your cancer risk, whilst increasing your omega-3 intake helps to balance this ratio and significantly reduces your cancer risk for a number of types of cancer.

A Japanese study on rats showed that wakame reduced breast-cancer cell proliferation. In another study, wakame root, known as mekabu, induced cell death in human hormone receptor negative (ER-/PR-) breast-cancer cells and suppressed mammary carcinogenesis. The extract of mekabu was administered in the rats' drinking water without any discernible toxicity.

Wakame may also help protect you from environmental exposure to dioxins. A study showed that wakame was effective in preventing the absorption and reabsorption of dioxin through the gut.

Whilst seaweed has been shown to be highly beneficial in a number of studies, one large study was delivered by mainstream media in a very alarmist fashion. They claimed that daily consumption of seaweed can greatly increase your risk of cancer.

The truth of the study was that out of 53,000 Japanese women (ranging in age from 40 to 69 years old) who ate seaweed daily over the course of 14 years, 134 women were diagnosed with thyroid cancer during the trial. The newspapers reported that this meant the women were 1.7 times more likely to develop cancer. This is not true. The research actually showed that they were 1.7 times more likely to develop thyroid cancer, which is quite rare. They entirely ignored the reduction in cancer rates of all other forms of cancer.

On balance, yes, thyroid cancer levels slightly increased to a 1 in 500 chance amongst postmenopausal women, but other cancers, such as breast cancer, (where you normally have a 1 in 8 chance of being diagnosed), were made considerably less likely.

By way of compromise, I would suggest that seaweed is still included as part of a healthy diet, but perhaps not daily.

With some varieties of seaweed having almost a third of their dry mass made up of micronutrients, they are hard to dismiss as a valid food source in the fight against cancer.

However, due to the pollution of the sea, some seaweeds can contain unacceptable levels of heavy metals, including arsenic. It is often down to where it is grown. You must also bear in mind that seaweed is not a good choice for people with thyroid disorders due to the high iodine levels. Equally, there is the possibility of high sodium content, which could affect blood pressure levels in those who are susceptible to high blood pressure.

Sesame seeds

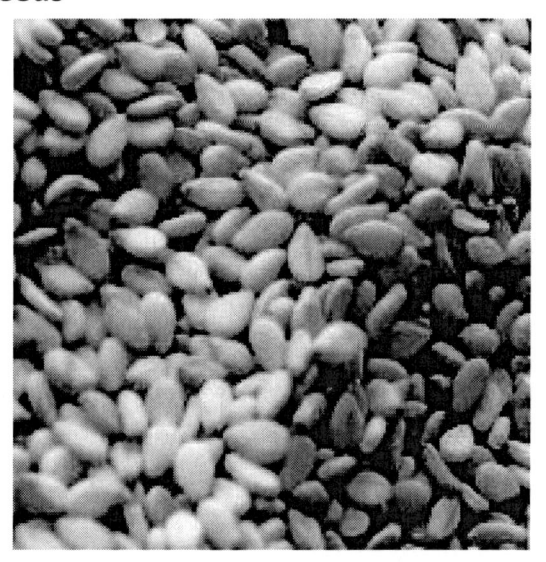

Sesame seeds are an excellent source of lignans, which have been shown to help fight hormonally driven cancers such as breast cancer or prostate cancer.

Other sources of lignans include brown rice, flaxseed and rye.

A cell study related to melanomas, discovered that when human malignant melanocytes were exposed to Sesame oil, the oil selectively inhibited the malignant melanoma growth.

In another study, using human lymphoid leukaemia cells, it was discovered that treatment with a sesame extract, called sesamolin, inhibited the growth of cells by triggering programmed cell death (apoptosis).

Sesame seeds are an easy addition to your diet, just sprinkle them on cereal, salads, soups, pasta, and more. They help form a delicious crunchy topping on cauliflower cheese, lasagne or anything else you might bake, containing cheese.

Soy

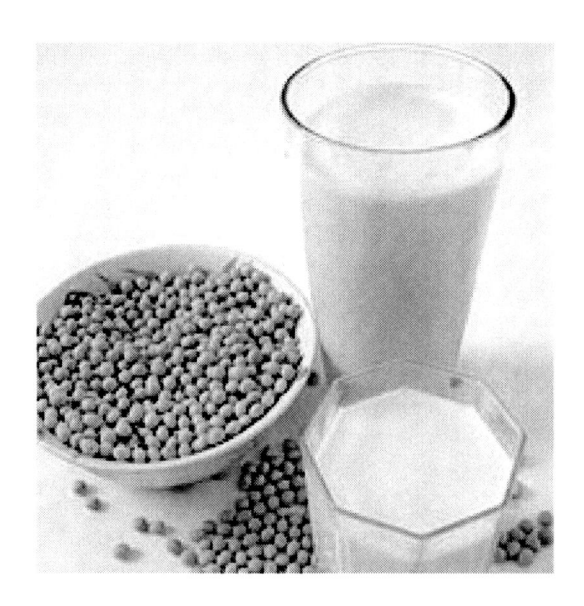

Soy products, including soy milk, soy beans, tofu, tempeh, miso, edamame, some veggie burgers and any food containing soy flour, are a little bit of an unknown quantity.

The confusion surrounds the fact that soy contains phytoestrogens, which are potentially able to mimic the effect of human oestrogen. This bears a relevance to hormonally-driven cancers such as prostate cancer, breast cancer and endometrial cancer.

On one hand, in the laboratory, phytoestrogens have been seen to stimulate the growth of breast cancer cells. On the other hand, diets high in soy-based products seem to indicate the reverse.

For example, a study reported in the Journal of the American Medical Association in 2009, based upon 5042 people in the

Shanghai breast cancer survival study, showed that soy significantly reduced the risk of both breast cancer recurrence and mortality. The only question was whether a study on Chinese women was relevant to Western women due to the differences in diet and lifestyle.

More recently, a study of 10,000 breast cancer survivors published in The American Journal of Clinical Nutrition, showed that women who consumed the greatest quantity of soy-based products had the lowest rates of cancer recurrence and mortality.

If you drill down into the issue in greater detail, you discover that the phytoestrogens from soy are from two kinds of isoflavones called genestein and diadzen. They can act like oestrogen in the body, however they are only a fraction as potent as the circulating oestrogen normally found in women.

So on the surface, you would assume that having more oestrogen-like compounds in the blood, which may trigger hormonally driven cancers, is bad. But looking at it another way, would you rather have potent human oestrogen binding with oestrogen receptors 100% of the time, or would you like a very weak version blocking up your oestrogen receptors some of the time, so that potent oestrogen cannot? This competition for your limited oestrogen receptors can give isoflavones "anti-oestrogen" properties.

Isoflavones have also been shown to help stop the formation of oestrogens in fat tissue, which is where your oestrogen comes from after menopause (unless you have hormone replacement therapy). They can also stimulate the production of a protein that binds oestrogen in the blood, making it less able to bind with your body's own oestrogen receptors. Combine this with anti-inflammatory and antioxidant properties and you have a solid argument for the consumption of soy.

On that basis, it is difficult to determine categorically whether soy does, or does not, trigger or fuel breast cancer.

My concerns are down to the fact that these studies were conducted on women who had already been diagnosed with breast cancer. They did not detail the effect of soy-based products on a population of healthy women.

There have been epidemiological studies on larger groups of healthy women. One notable study combine the data from 14 different epidemiologic studies. They discovered that in Asian countries, the women who consumed the greatest amounts of isoflavones had a 24% lower risk of developing breast cancer than those who consumed the least. However, there was no obvious association in Western countries at all.

This is because in Western countries, those women considered to have the "highest" levels of consumption actually ate less soy-based products than those Asian women with the least consumption. "High" consumption for Asian women was the equivalent of four portions per day of soy products, whereas "high" consumption for Western women was less than half a portion per day.

Equally, the possible impact of consuming a soy-based diet through puberty and breast development, cannot be taken into consideration in a typical Western population, because the consequences of this impact are unknown.

Like many foods, soy products in moderation are unlikely to do significant harm, and in the case of breast cancer survivors, an increase in soy (albeit based on limited data) seems to reduce your risk of recurrence or mortality from the condition.

It is down to each individual, and the advice from their doctor, to determine whether or not they will include soy in their diet.

As a general rule of thumb, when it comes to food, the closer a product is to its raw state, the better it is for your health. Soy takes around three days of processing to make it edible. So I am slightly averse to soy on an instinctive level, but I cannot argue with the data for those women who have already been diagnosed with breast cancer.

Equally, for men who have been diagnosed with prostate cancer (the fourth most common cancer in the world), I would seriously advise you to look into the benefits of soy. Asian countries have a much lower level of prostate cancer, and studies have shown that when Asian men start living in the US, they have a tenfold increase in the rates of prostate cancer.

In cell culture studies, the isoflavone genistein has been shown to inhibit prostate cancer cell growth and trigger programmed cell death. It has also been shown in other studies to increase the effectiveness of radiation in killing prostate cancer cells. In rodent studies, high soy diets were linked to a reduction in the number of prostate tumours, an increase in the rate of cancer cell death, a decrease in tumour blood vessel development and researchers noted that the disease was typically less aggressive compared with control groups.

Spinach

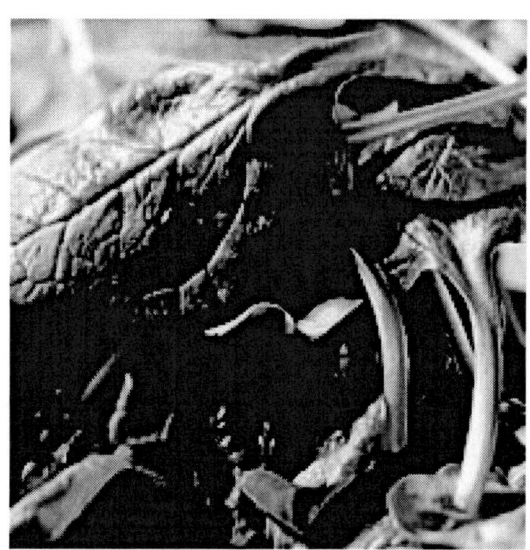

Spinach has long been known as a source of iron and folic acid and other phytochemicals. Research has identified at least 13

different flavonoid compounds within spinach that act as antioxidants and anti-cancer agents.

Interestingly, just like beetroot, spinach has been shown in clinical research to make muscles more efficient, by reducing the oxygen they need to perform exercise. Within just three days of eating the equivalent of a plate of spinach per day, volunteers reduced their oxygen requirements for exercise by 5%. This is because the nitrates within the spinach enable cells to greatly increase the rate at which they absorb oxygen, but also made the energy conversion process within the mitochondria of cells more efficient.

In vitro studies, using human liver cancer cells, colon cancer cells and breast cancer cells, have shown that spinach has the highest antiproliferative effect, compared with other vegetables.

A notable study on cervical cancer showed that the retinoids found in spinach had chemotherapeutic chemopreventive potential.

A study on gallbladder cancer discovered that the greater the spinach consumption, the lower the risk of gallbladder cancer.

And finally, a National Cancer Institute study showed that a higher intake of lutein and zeaxanthin containing foods, including spinach, corresponds to a lower risk of non-Hodgkin's lymphoma (NHL).

Strawberries

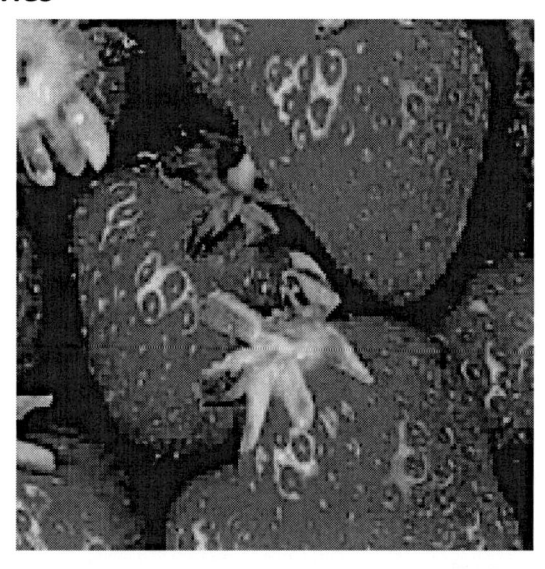

Strawberries are a rich source of vitamin C and iron. They are also an excellent source of a soluble fibre called pectin, which helps your body eliminate harmful cholesterol. Several studies have highlighted that strawberries could be a valuable weapon in combating conditions such as heart disease, anaemia and even cancer.

Recent study data presented by the American Association for Cancer Research in 2011 showed that in both rats and humans, freeze-dried strawberries consumed daily, slowed the progression of oesophageal cancer, and prevented precancerous lesions in the oesophagus progressing into cancer.

Oesophageal cancer is the third most common gastrointestinal cancer, and the sixth most frequent cause of cancer death in the world. Just 60g of dried strawberries per day were used in the human participants for six months.

Other studies, including one study conducted by Harvard researchers have shown that strawberries can have an impact on numerous types of cancer - from leukaemia cells through to colon cancer cells, through to breast cancer cells and cervical cancer cells.

Strawberries are rich in ellagic acid, which is believed to be an oestrogen blocker, so this may be a potent tool in the fight against breast cancer.

The only drawback is that strawberries are one of the most pesticide-laden fruits due to modern farming methods, so choosing organic strawberries is highly recommended. They are sweeter, higher in antioxidants and don't contain harmful contaminants. Organic strawberries were found to be more effective in cancer studies, due to their higher levels of antioxidants.

Sunflower seeds

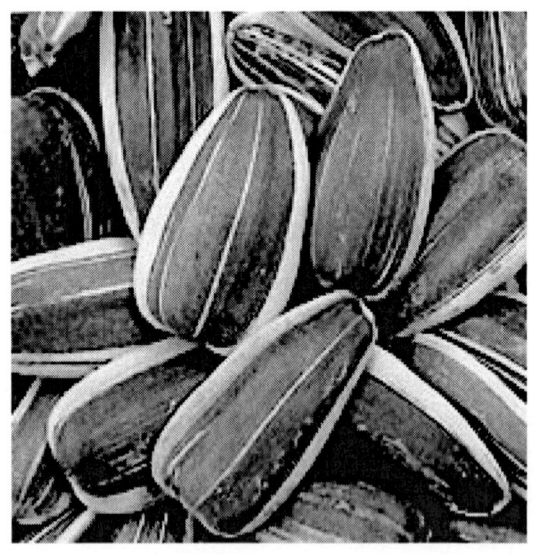

Sunflower seeds contain vitamin B1, vitamin E, folate, copper, selenium, magnesium and a range of phytosterols.

Studies on mice with stage II skin cancer have demonstrated that sunflower oil reduced papillomas by 20 to 40% compared with control groups.

Numerous studies have also shown that sunflower oil decreases levels of LDL (bad) cholesterol, thereby reducing the risk of heart disease.

Sunflower seeds are inexpensive and can be purchased already removed from their shells and ready to eat, making them a convenient snack food.

Sweet Potatoes

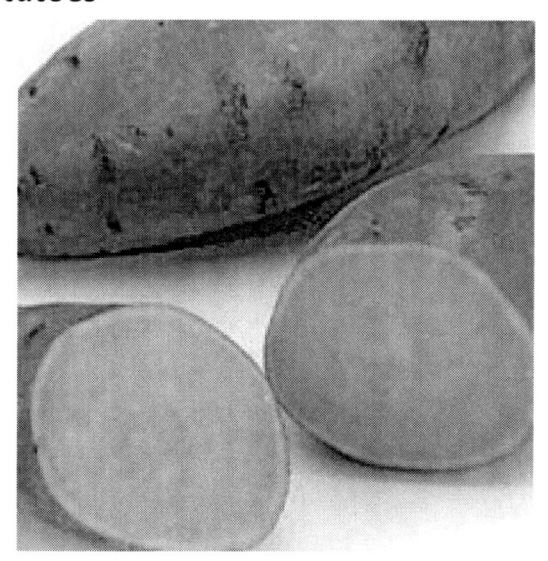

Whilst sweet potatoes are sometimes used as an alternative to conventional potatoes due to their high levels of carbohydrates, they are far superior in terms of their nutritional value. In addition to some protein, vitamin E and vitamin C, they contain very high levels of carotenoids, such as beta-carotene.

There is a large volume of data linking the consumption of sweet potatoes to a reduction in cancer risk.

As little as 100g of sweet potato per day has been found to dramatically reduce the risk of lung cancer.

Beta-carotene, from sweet potatoes, is stored in the fat layer of our skin and therefore also helps to protect us from damage from the ultraviolet rays produced by the sun.

A study on rats showed that the addition of purple sweet potatoes inhibited colorectal cancer. A study involving diagnosed cases of gallbladder cancer showed that sweet potatoes were among the vegetables that offered the greatest protective benefits. The Japanese study of 100,000 people over a ten-year period discovered that sweet potato consumption was consistent with a significant decrease in kidney cancer risk.

The high levels of vitamin B6 in sweet potato also help us to regulate our blood sugar levels, which is good for preventing the premature ageing of tissues due to excess blood sugar. It also helps us to prevent mood swings and relieve depression.

Tomatoes

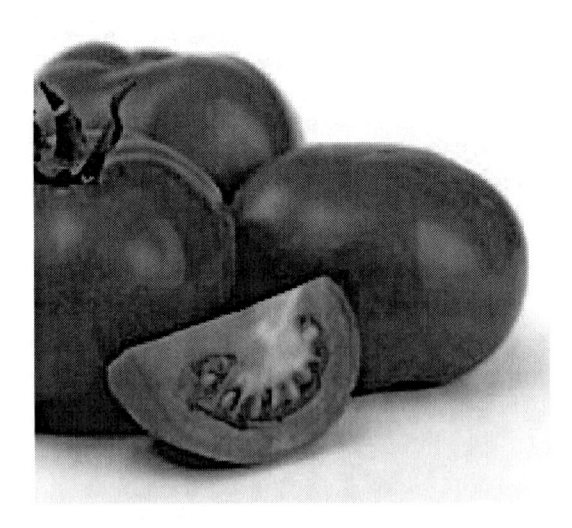

Tomatoes contain lycopene, an antioxidant with strong anti-cancer effects. For absorption, remember that they must be eaten with a small amount of oil, as in tomato sauce, tomato ketchup, or a fresh tomato salad with a little cold-pressed olive oil. This is because lycopene is oil soluble and needs the oil to carry it into your body whilst being digested.

Watermelon and pink grapefruit also contain lycopene, although at a lower concentration.

Studies have shown that tomatoes can have an impact on a range of different types of cancer, including colorectal cancer, ovarian cancer and prostate cancer.

Most notably, in a study on individuals due for a prostatectomy, those individuals who consumed tomato sauce on a daily basis in the three weeks leading up to their surgery, displayed a significant decrease in DNA damage to prostate tissues, and had a much higher rate of programmed cell death.

Other studies have found significant correlation between high plasma levels of lycopene and reduced risk of prostate cancer.

Power Combination: combine broccoli with tomatoes. Tomatoes are a potent source of lycopene. When lycopene was combined with the glycosinolates in broccoli, animal studies showed a tomato/broccoli combination was able to reduce tumour size by up to 52%.

Turmeric

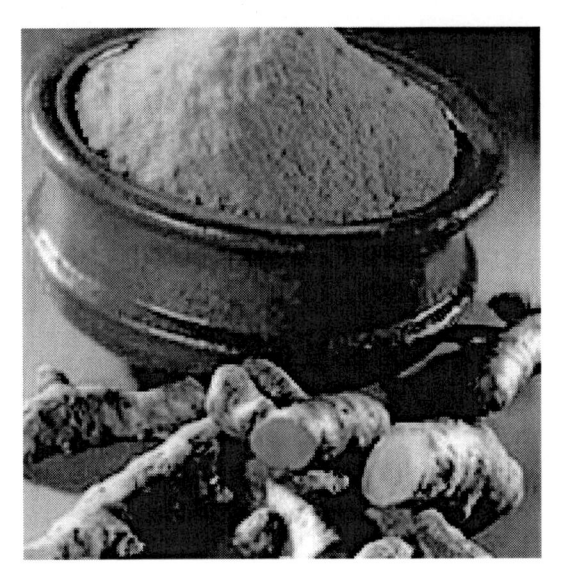

Turmeric is often found in curries and other Indian dishes. The active ingredient within turmeric is a phytochemical called curcumin, and it is this ingredient that gives curry its bright yellow colouring.

Curcumin has strong antioxidant properties, along with being an anti-inflammatory, antifungal and anti-viral agent.

A study conducted by the University of Texas, discovered that in cancer cells treated with curcumin, growth was inhibited and an increase in programmed cell death occurred.

Animal studies have shown that when turmeric was used, skin tumour occurrence was reduced by 87% (in comparison with the control group), and tumour size was reduced by 30%.

In mice studies, mice with breast cancer showed a substantially reduced spread of cancer to their lungs when curcumin was added to their diets.

A relatively small human trial was carried out on patients with precancerous polyps. They were treated with curcumin for a period of six months, which had the effect of reducing the average number of polyps by 60% and reduced the average size of each polyp by 50%. This is significant in terms of the potential reduction of colon cancer.

Other research has shown that curcumin reduces the expression of prostate cancer genes, and in animal studies curcumin reduced the tumour volume and quantity of nodules in treated animals, compared with control groups.

Not only has turmeric been found to have both anti-inflammatory and cancer fighting properties, it has also been discovered that turmeric can be used to suppress the biological mechanisms that trigger inflammation in tendon diseases. The only difficulty is getting a sufficient dose. There is only 3.6g of curcumin in 100g of curry powder.

One additional factor that is worthy of note, is that curcumin also inhibits a bacteria that is linked to the vast majority of stomach ulcers called Helicobacter pylori. Many individuals with acid reflux and indigestion may have an undiagnosed Helicobacter pylori infection in their stomachs, and studies have shown that such infections are very likely to cause stomach ulcers. Beyond that, there is a strong link between stomach ulcers and stomach cancer. Therefore, by targeting the cause, you also target the symptom.

Certainly, if you have a stomach ulcer, you should demand that your doctor tests you for H. pylori, as a simple course of antibiotics could eliminate the cause of your ulcer and drastically reduce your likelihood of getting stomach cancer.

Walnuts

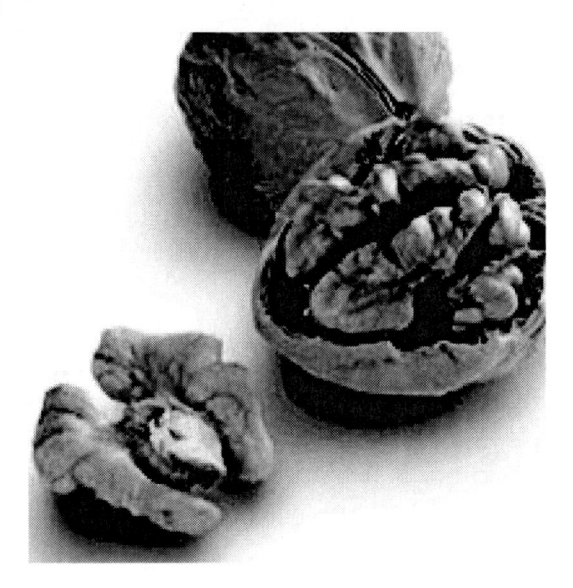

Walnuts have the highest levels of omega-3 essential fatty acids found in any nut. They are also a rich source of vitamin E.

A recent US study showed that daily consumption of walnuts cut the risk of breast cancer in half in laboratory mice. The human dose equivalent would be around 2 ounces of walnuts per day. In addition, the tumours diagnosed within the group consuming walnuts, (along with their existing diet), were significantly smaller and less numerous.

The researchers stated "these reductions are particularly important when you consider that the mice were genetically programmed to develop cancer at a high rate." "We were able to reduce the risk for cancer even in the presence of a pre-existing genetic mutation".

The researchers were clear that there are multiple compounds within walnuts that reduce the risk of cancer or slow its growth, including omega-3 essential fatty acids and vitamin E.

Further genetic analysis concluded that the walnut-containing diet changed the activity of multiple genes that are associated with breast cancer in both mice and humans, so the data should be relevant to human breast cancer. This just highlights the vital role that nutrition can play in cancer prevention.

Water

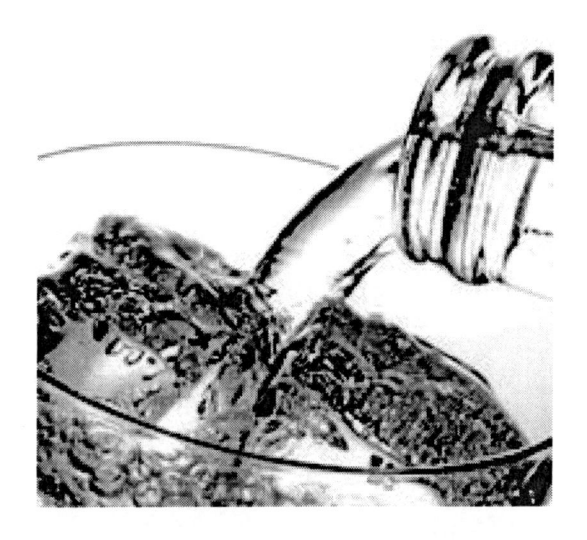

Water is essential for almost every process within our bodies. In fact your body comprises over 70% water. Drinking plenty of water every day increases your cellular hydration, rehydrating the skin and helping your body to eliminate toxins. Try to avoid flavoured water, because it is loaded with artificial sweeteners or sugar.

You should also be aware that the mechanism that triggers thirst deteriorates as we age, so you should not wait until you are thirsty before you drink. Try to consume 2 litres of water each day.

Dehydration can cause constipation, can impair brain function and can lead to greater inflammation of mucous membranes during times of illness.

The one caveat I would add is that filtered water is the best option. Mineral water is great in theory, but the plasticisers, leaching out of the plastic bottle it comes in, detract from its appeal.

I use a water filter system with 13 stages, that helps to remove heavy metals, pesticides, bacteria and many other unwanted substances. It finishes by re-mineralising the water and balancing its pH to be more alkaline by using coral. You can purchase them from eBay for the equivalent of around £90 or $150, but it will produce water for over a year on a single filter.

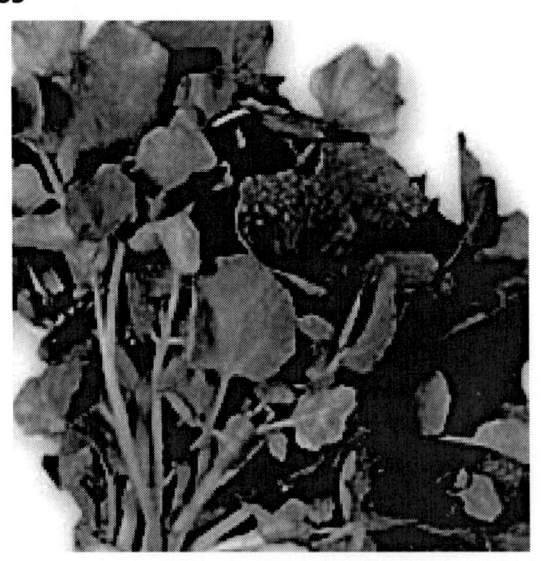

Watercress

Watercress is a super food. Gram for gram, it contains more vitamin C than oranges, more iron than spinach, more quercetin than broccoli or tomatoes. It also contains folic acid, calcium, iron and beta-carotene.

Watercress extracts have been shown to inhibit the growth of breast cancer cells. Researchers, writing in the British Journal of Nutrition, believe that it is due to the isothiocyanates found in watercress. This belief is based upon other epidemiological studies that show that people who consume watercress and other isothiocyanate-rich vegetables, including cabbage and broccoli, have a lower risk of developing cancer.

A pilot study of breast cancer survivors were given a diet including watercress. Scientists discovered that six hours after consuming the watercress leaves, blood samples showed a drop in the activity of a molecule called 4E binding protein 1 (4E-BP1), which is believed necessary for the cancer's survival.

Of course, more in-depth studies are required, but adding watercress to your diet is a simple process. Add it to salads, sandwiches, soups and as a garnish with any other meal.

Whey

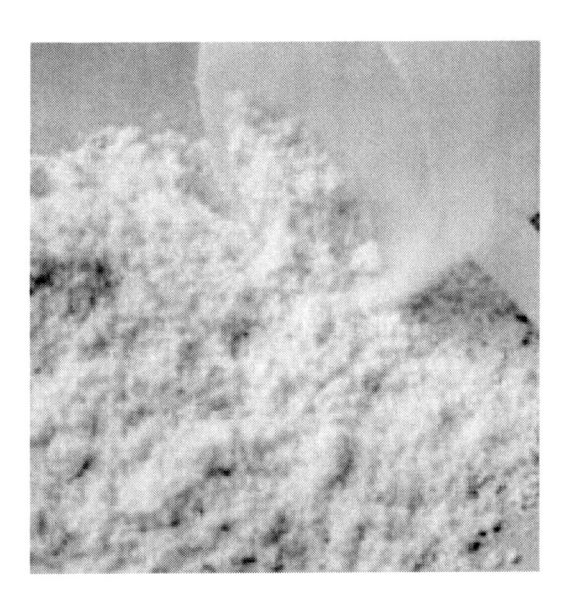

Whey protein is a natural byproduct of the cheesemaking process. It typically comes in the form of a powdered supplement, available in most health food outlets, or for purchase online.

As a supplement, whey protein is available as whey protein concentrate and whey protein isolates. Isolates contain in excess of 90% protein, with little or no fat, and no lactose. Many people who have allergies to dairy, have a sensitivity to casein, which is a larger milk protein, and they do not actually have a problem with whey protein.

Whey protein contains branched-chain amino acids (BCAAs), which are the building blocks needed for the development and repair of muscles and other tissues.

Whey protein has a number of fascinating properties, and research has gone into its benefit in the treatment of cardiovascular disease, osteoporosis, hepatitis B, HIV and cancer.

Whey protein boosts your immune system, adds to your muscle mass, prevents muscle wastage, increases bone density and stimulates the body to produce cholecystokinin (CCK), a hormone that is released after eating to give a sense of satiety. This has been shown to help with weight loss by suppressing hunger urges. (Almonds do the same thing).

Studies have shown that whey protein inhibits the growth of breast cancer cells. Another clinical study showed the regression of certain types of cancer when patients were given 30g of whey protein per day.

Whey protein contains a high level of the amino acid cysteine, which enables your body to produce a cell protector called glutathione. This water-soluble antioxidant protects your cells from the harmful effects of free radicals and it helps to neutralise toxins including heavy metals, peroxides, carcinogens and more.

Animal studies have shown that whey protein increases glutathione levels more than any other form of protein, including soy protein.

A number of diseases, including atherosclerosis, Alzheimer's, Parkinson's, AIDS and cancer are associated with reduced glutathione levels, and studies with whey protein have helped to reverse this imbalance. For example a study of HIV positive men showed that whey protein supplements could restore their glutathione levels, with two out of three men able to return to an ideal weight.

Cancer cells can be difficult to treat because they often have a much higher and more protective level of glutathione than normal cells, and normal cells can be depleted of glutathione during times of disease. Therefore, when chemotherapy takes place, the cancer cells are more resistant than normal tissue.

According to research published in Anti Cancer Research 1996, whey protein has the interesting property of reducing the glutathione levels in cancer cells, whilst simultaneously increasing the glutathione levels (and therefore antioxidant protection) in healthy noncancerous cells.

Whey protein also contains lactoferrin, which is an antioxidant that helps to mop up free iron molecules in the intestines. It is so effective, that it has been shown to inhibit the growth of iron-dependent bacteria, and can inhibit the growth of pathogenic bacteria and yeast. It also helps defend against uncontrolled oxidative damage caused by iron free radicals. This is excellent if you eat red meat.

Overall, I believe that whey protein is a solid addition to your diet for the immune boosting, cancer cell inhibiting, and gut health properties. However, make sure you purchase whey protein isolates and not just whey protein concentrate that may contain higher levels of lactose and fat.

Equally, I would recommend whey protein from outside of the US (unless it is organic), because over 80% of genetically modified grains and corn go into animal feed in the US, and you run the risk of indirect consumption of these harmful and potentially carcinogenic products. Please see the section on GMO (genetically modified organism) foods, under "Foods to Avoid".

If you would like to see a list of suppliers who provide certified organic whey from non-GMO, grass-fed cattle free from hormone injections and anti-biotics, which is cold processed with no artificial sweeteners, please visit:

http://www.CancerUncensored.com/organic-whey

Whole Grains

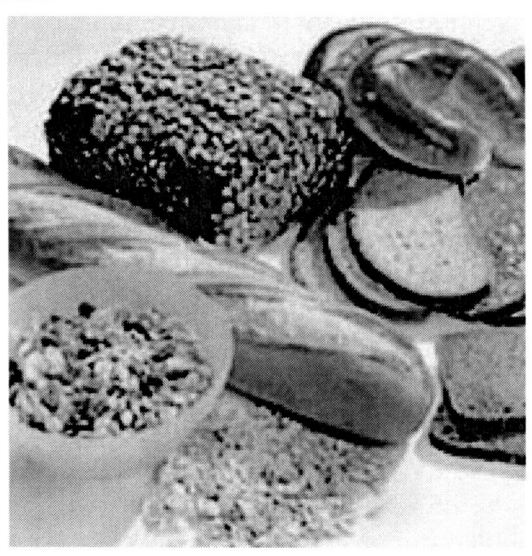

(Please also see the section on "Foods to Avoid" for issues related to wheat)

Whole grains have long been associated with significant improvements to heart health and cholesterol levels. However, indications of a reduced risk of cancer are a more recent discovery.

According to the British Medical Journal in 2011, cereals and whole grains could reduce the risk of developing colorectal cancer.

Researchers from Imperial College London revealed that for every 10g of additional fibre intake per day from whole grain sources, the risk of bowel cancer decreased by 10%.

There has long been a relationship between eating fibre and whole grains and the reduction in risk of cardiovascular disease, but cancer has been harder to study.

This study involved the collection of data from over 25 previous studies, which meant that the data analysed was from almost 2,000,000 people.

Their definition of whole grain foods included wholegrain breads, brown rice, cereals, oatmeal and porridge. Previous studies have shown a reduced risk from a high intake of fruit and vegetables, (that also contain dietary fibre), but the researchers did not wish to acknowledge it because other chemical factors would also be at play.

As you will see in the chapter relating to foods to avoid, I highlight certain risk factors connected with modern wheat (which has undergone a whole series of modifications since the 1950s). However, there are a wide range of different whole grains to choose from, such as brown rice, rye, quinoa, oats, barley, amaranth and more.

The advantage of wholegrain foods, are that they contain all of the essential parts of the entire seed. Refined grains, which would include white flour, have had many components stripped away, such as a high proportion of the protein and as many as 17 different key nutrients.

Foods to Avoid

The following foods have been determined to increase your risk of cancer. On that basis, you should seriously consider cutting them out of your diet, particularly if you have already been diagnosed with cancer.

Of course, there is always the balance between life expectancy and enjoyment while you are here, so you must strike your own balance.

Alcohol

Alcohol is now the third leading contributor to premature death and is linked to the deaths of 1.8 million people worldwide every year.

It compromises your ability to intake nutrition (by reducing the bacterial population of your gut), it can have a negative effect on your immune system, and being a solvent, it is able to promote genetic change. On this basis, almost any illness you can get is made more likely by a high-level consumption of alcohol, and, by the same token, any illness you may already have is typically made worse by it.

As a result, alcohol has been implicated in increasing your risk of cancer, heart disease, stroke, obesity, infertility, osteoporosis and more.

Alcoholic drinks such as red wine, are often viewed as being less harmful, due to high levels of antioxidants and phytochemicals, but the exact same health benefits can be obtained by eating red grapes.

Of course, long-term studies on alcohol consumption indicate that low levels of consumption pose minimal risk to your health, so your consumption of alcohol is a personal choice.

In a study of over 105,000 women, researchers discovered that those who consumed 3 to 6 glasses of wine per week were 15% more likely to receive a diagnosis of breast cancer. Those women who drank fewer than three drinks per week, did not statistically increase their risk at all. On that basis, the occasional glass of wine or cocktail was not an issue, it was the repeated ongoing consumption of alcohol that triggered the increase in risk.

If you have already been diagnosed with cancer, I would recommend not consuming alcohol at all.

Artificial sweeteners

Also known as sugar substitutes, artificial sweeteners are alternatives to table sugar (sucrose), that are used to sweeten foods and beverages.

Artificial sweeteners are typically many times sweeter than sugar, which means that only tiny amounts of them need to be used to recreate the same level of sweetness. The supposed "advantage" of these sweeteners is that generally, your body cannot utilise them as calories, which means that they do not contribute to your daily calorie intake.

Artificial sweeteners are regulated by the US Food and Drug Administration (FDA). The Food Additives Amendment to the Food, Drug and Cosmetic Act 1958, requires the FDA to approve food additives, including some artificial sweeteners, but this legislation doesn't apply to products considered to be "generally recognised as safe".

Between 1999 and 2004, there were more than 6000 new products launched that contained artificial sweeteners. As a result, it is estimated that 15% of the Western world are regularly consuming artificial sweeteners, with or without their knowledge.

There have been persistent questions regarding the safety of artificial sweeteners since early studies showed that a combination of cyclamate and saccharin resulted in laboratory animals forming bladder cancer.

A variety of sweeteners have caused concern, but the official FDA position is that there is no "clear evidence" that artificial sweeteners have an association with cancer in humans.

Studies on saccharin in the 1970s demonstrated an increase in urinary bladder cancer in rats (particularly male rats), which prompted Congress to mandate that food containing saccharin bore the label "Use of this product may be hazardous to your health. This product contains saccharin, which has been determined to cause cancer in laboratory animals".

However, further research into the mechanism by which the saccharin caused cancer indicated that it was safe for humans, so saccharin was delisted in 2000 from the Report on Carcinogens Published by the US National Toxicology Program.

Aspartame, which is provided under several different brand names (including NutraSweet® and Equal®), is found in a range of food and drinks, from chewing gum to cola, and from breakfast cereals to yoghurt. It is around 200 times sweeter than table sugar, and if it isn't listed as aspartame, it is listed as E951.

Aspartame has had a rocky journey through its approval process with the FDA with some considerable controversy and conflicts of interest.

It was approved for use in dry foods in 1974, based upon 168 studies presented by G.D. Searle & Company, (otherwise known as Searle), the pharmaceutical company who owned the patent on aspartame. However, a petition for a public hearing was filed, citing safety concerns. It was asserted that unreported medical treatments may have affected the study outcomes and that there were discrepancies in reported data. The FDA Commissioner in 1975, Alexander Schmidt, agreed to investigate alleged improprieties in safety studies for aspartame, which resulted in the FDA placing a stay on the aspartame approval.

Schmidt openly criticised the Searle studies as being "... at best... sloppy and suffering from... a pattern of conduct which compromises the scientific integrity of the studies."

US attorney Samuel Skinner was requested to "open a grand jury investigation into whether two of Searle's aspartame studies had been falsified or were incomplete".

If you were cynical, you might wonder why Skinner withdrew from the case after he was given a job offer from Searle's Chicago-based lawyers Sidley & Austin. The resultant delay caused by Skinner's removal from the case meant that the statute of limitations on the charges against Searle expired. This meant a grand jury was never convened.

The interim U.S. attorney for Chicago, William Conlon, who held the position in transition, would not convene a grand jury either. As luck might have it, he also landed himself a nice new job at Searle's law firm.

In 1977 and 1978 a panel of pathologists reviewed 15 aspartame studies by Searle. They concluded that although minor inconsistencies were found they would not have affected the conclusions of the studies.

But in 1980, a public board of enquiry heard testimony from Prof John Olney, who claimed that aspartame could cause brain cancer, including in developing foetuses. The board declared that further study data was required and revoked the approval of aspartame.

In 1981, FDA Commissioner Arthur Hull Hayes sought advice from a panel of FDA scientists and a lawyer who presented arguments both for and against the approval of aspartame. Arthur Hull Hayes decided to approve the use of aspartame anyway. There were a number of objections, all of which were denied. If you were cynical, you might wonder why a year later, Arthur Hull Hayes left the FDA for a nice new job at Searle's public relations firm Burson-Marsteller, acting as a senior medical adviser. Burson-Marsteller promoted NutraSweet® for Searle.

In 1987, an investigation was carried out by the US Government Accountability Office. Despite a survey of 67 scientists who had expertise on the topic, (12 of which had major concerns about aspartame safety and 26 were somewhat concerned), aspartame was allowed to retain its approval.

Concerns regarding aspartame's safety were raised again in 1996, after it was noticed that there was a significant increase in brain cancer over the period since the introduction of aspartame. These claims were later dismissed, because this increasing trend in brain cancer could be traced back to a time slightly earlier than the launch of aspartame.

A psychologist at Northeastern Ohio University's College of medicine, Ralph G. Walton published an analysis of prior aspartame research. It showed that whilst industry-funded studies had found no safety concerns, 84 out of the 92 independent studies did show safety concerns. A rebuttal soon followed by the Aspartame Information Service, provided by a primary producer and supplier of aspartame, criticising Walton's research.

However, several studies spanning 2005-2007 by the Cesare Maltoni Cancer Research Center of the European Ramazzini Foundation of Oncology and Environmental Sciences, showed significantly more leukaemias, lymphomas and breast cancers in rats fed with high doses of aspartame. Doses that were consistent with supposedly safe amounts in humans.

There were some inconsistencies in the data, which largely related to the fact that increasing the level of aspartame didn't necessarily increase the number of cancer cases.

Currently, aspartame is widely used by the food and drinks industry and is approved by the FDA, but that doesn't necessarily mean that aspartame is entirely safe. After all, aspartame breaks down into methanol, which subsequently breaks down into formaldehyde, a known carcinogen and neurotoxin. (Although this is supposed to be at such a low level that it is not considered toxic).

H.J. Roberts MD, in his book "Aspartame Disease: An Ignored Epidemic", covers numerous negative health consequences relating to ingesting aspartame. According to Dr Roberts, by 1988, 80% of the complaints to the FDA about food additives related to aspartame products. Some of the symptoms include abdominal pain, headaches, vomiting and nausea, changes in mood, dizziness, fatigue, memory loss, diarrhoea, joint pain, depression, slurred speech, anxiety attacks and more.

In terms of independent studies, there is some data that is difficult to ignore. In one study relating to migraines, in randomised double-blind placebo controlled studies, migraine sufferers had headaches more frequently and more severely when they consumed aspartame.

In another study related to the effect of aspartame on depression, the study had to be cut short due to the severity of the reactions. It appeared that individuals with mood disorders were particularly sensitive to the effects of aspartame.

Aspartame may have some serious skeletons in the closet where its approval is concerned, and when several key players in the approval process end up with nice new jobs, all linked to the biggest beneficiary of the approval, you have to wonder who you can trust.

(See also the GMO section to see evidence of key FDA officials swapping between the FDA payroll and the applicant's payroll after key decisions have been made about potentially dangerous products. Searle was acquired by Monsanto in 1985, and Monsanto is central to the current GMO-related cancer controversies. If aspartame wasn't controversial enough, it is now being manufactured using genetically modified bacteria, combining two of the most controversial and dangerous aspects of the food industry).

"The thing that bugs me is that people think the FDA is protecting them. It isn't. What the FDA is doing and what the public thinks it's doing are as different as night and day." - Herbert Lay, former Commissioner of the FDA.

Aspartame is now a financial juggernaut within the food industry, and to remove it would affect thousands of products and open all manner of avenues for litigation. So unless the evidence (and public pressure) is overwhelming, I do not see the classification changing any time soon. Just look at how long it took to determine that cigarette smoking is dangerous.

The light at the end of the tunnel is that various governments and regulatory bodies have now looked at banning aspartame from the food supply. Including, in March 2009, the California OEHHA, who identified aspartame as a chemical for consultation by its Carcinogen Identification Committee.

In 2007, the UK supermarket chains Marks & Spencer, Sainsbury's and Asda (a UK subsidiary of Walmart) announced that they would no longer use aspartame in their own label products.

In 2009, Woolworths announced it was removing aspartame from its own brand foods.

In 2010, the British Food Standards Agency, launched an investigation after receiving reports of side effects from aspartame. Unsurprisingly, the study has not yet been concluded because the FSA are having trouble finding enough volunteers.

In 2011, The European Food Safety Authority (EFSA) commenced a full re-evaluation of aspartame, the results of which should be available by May 2013. This will include previously unpublished scientific data.

Other artificial sweeteners include a acesulfame potassium (or acesulfame K), also known as Sweet One®, Sunnett® and ACK, sucralose, also known as Splenda®, and Neotame®, which is similar to aspartame.

Acesulfame K contains methylene chloride, which is a known carcinogen. The effects of long-term exposure to methylene chloride include nausea, depression, headaches, mental confusion, visual disturbances, kidney effects, liver problems and cancer in humans. There's been very little long-term testing to ensure this product's safety, and at this moment in time the FDA do not require these tests to be carried out.

Neotame® is chemically similar to aspartame, which could indicate the same risks. Unfortunately the studies that have been carried out on it do not address long-term health implications. Whilst the website for Neotame® claim over 100 scientific studies to support its safety, the studies are not easily available for public consumption.

You would assume that sucralose would have a better track record, but unfortunately as Dr. Mercola highlights, as of 2006:

"Only six human trials have been published on sucralose. Of these six trials, only two of the trials were completed and published before the FDA approved sucralose for human consumption. The two published trials had a grand total of 36 total human subjects…The longest trial at this time had lasted only four days and looked at sucralose in relation to tooth decay, not human tolerance."

The final nail in the coffin for artificial sweeteners, is the fact that studies have shown that increased consumption of artificial sweeteners is linked to weight gain. This completely defeats their purpose!

The American Cancer Society studied 78,694 women over a one-year period and found that as much as 7.1% more of the women using artificial sweeteners gained weight in comparison with those who did not use artificial sweeteners.

The San Antonio heart study, conducted upon 3,682 adults over an eight-year period, showed that those individuals who consumed more artificial sweeteners had a higher BMI (body mass index). The greater the artificial sweetener consumption, the greater the BMI.

It is not entirely clear whether the artificial sweeteners triggered appetite, or whether the sweeteners encourage your body to store more of the food you eat.

Researchers at Liverpool University discovered that artificial sweeteners still trigger the same receptors in your gut which initiate the release of hormones that help your body absorb the sugar within the food you have just eaten. As a result, food combined with artificial sweeteners were more readily absorbed and stored as fat.

Researchers at the University of Texas San Antonio discovered that artificial sweeteners increased cravings. After following 600 participants, aged 25 to 64, over an eight-year period, they discovered that those individuals who consumed one diet soda per day were 65% more likely to be overweight than those who drank none. In fact, the participants who consumed diet drinks had a greater chance of becoming overweight than those who drank regular soda / soft drinks!

Ordinarily, consuming sugar triggers a release of leptin, which signals to our brains that we've satisfied our hunger. But artificial sweeteners do not trigger this release.

Artificial sweeteners also interfere with our usual blood sugar control mechanisms, including our insulin response. When you consume an artificially sweetened diet drink, it does not contribute to your blood sugar levels. However, it does trigger a surge of insulin, even though you haven't actually consumed any usable calories.

This dump of insulin contributes to your likelihood of type II diabetes and obesity, either by adding extra load on to your pancreas, or else by triggering a greater insulin response when you combine the diet drink with food, thereby storing more of the food you just washed down with the artificially sweetened drink.

To avoid artificial sweeteners, look out for any foods that say "diet", "sugarfree", or "reduced sugar". In particular, read the labels of diet drinks, chewing gum, yoghurts, crisps / chips, flavoured water, cereals, drink powders, and some low-fat products, such as cakes, where manufacturers try to improve the flavour with artificial sweeteners.

You should also be on your guard against sneaky marketing tricks used on food labelling. Aspartame is being rebranded as "AminoSweet" to give it the impression of being natural and safe. But it is still the same dubious product, so do not be hoodwinked.

Whilst I wouldn't necessarily advocate table sugar, I would ALWAYS choose it over artificial sweeteners, if honey wasn't an option. After all, a whole teaspoon of sugar only contains 16 calories, and it isn't neurotoxic.

Caffeine / Coffee

A study conducted by researchers from Harvard University and Tokyo Women's Medical University, following over 38,000 women over the course of 10 years, has shown that drinking more than 4 cups of coffee per day increased the risk of breast cancer by 68%.

The researchers also discovered that a high caffeine diet increased the likelihood of larger tumour formation by 79%, (defined as tumours greater than 2cm).

However, research published in the journal Cancer Research, showed that in a study of 112,000 individuals, those people consuming an average of 2 cups of coffee per day or greater, decreased the likelihood of developing basal cell carcinoma, a slow-growing, but common form of skin cancer.

These studies indicate that the matter is perhaps more complex. Perhaps caffeine has benefits, whereas coffee has risks, or vice versa, because the consumption of coffee appears to have both positive and negative effects were cancer is concerned.

The root problem may be that the complex structure of the amino acid in Coffee causes a binding reaction with many important minerals, which chelates them out of the body. Coffee has been linked to fibroids, polyps and cysts in women and prostate issues in men. It also contributes to osteoporosis and arthritis.

Given that breast cancer is likely to affect one in eight Western women within their lifetime, and that it has a significantly more concerning prognosis than basal cell carcinoma (which rarely kills and almost never spreads to other parts of the body), I would suggest a reduction in coffee intake. If you do continue to use caffeine, get it from green tea, which has many other health benefits.

Processed meats

Meats that have been preserved by curing, salting, smoking or by adding chemical preservatives have been shown to increase your risk of bowel, stomach, oesophagus and mouth cancers. Burnt or charred meat may also increase the cancer risk.

Studies show that in Europe, daily consumption of 50g of cured meat per day increases your risk of colorectal cancer by approximately 30%.

Meats, such as hot dogs, bacon, ham, gammon, sausages, cold cuts, often contain nitrites, which are chemical preservatives. Nitrites, whilst necessary for killing the deadly botulism bacterium, have been shown to increase your risk of stomach and bowel cancer. Better to avoid nitrites in cured meats altogether, but if you don't, then try to consume them with beetroot on the side (as part of a salad) or as beetroot juice. See the Beetroot section for more details on how it counteracts the harm from nitrites.

According to animal studies, the cancer risk of red meat (not processed or cured meat) appears to be linked with heminic iron, which is what makes red meat red. One way of reducing the risk would be to eat a source of calcium along with red meat, which lowers the absorption of iron from food. For example, eating yoghurt or a piece of cheese after consuming steak.

Alternatively, add a source of lactoferrin to your diet, such as whey protein, because this can mop up free iron molecules.

In Europe, studies show that daily consumption of red meat totalling 80g per day or greater, increases your colorectal cancer risk by around 20%.

The China-Cornell-Oxford Project, often referred to as the China Study, a 20-year study that began in 1983 and was conducted jointly by the Chinese Academy of Preventive Medicine, Cornell University, and the University of Oxford, concluded that the consumption of animal protein may be the single biggest dietary factor in cutting short our life-span through a range of Western diseases. So if you are serious about your health, going vegetarian has a lot to be said for it.

Animal products account for as much as 40% of the diet of the average American.

Many people do not go vegetarian through concerns that they cannot get "complete" protein from plant sources. However, this is a fallacy. Most plants contain all of the essential amino acids, but they may be low in a particular kind. Low, but not missing. By combining foods with a different amino acid profile, such as beans or legumes with rice, (as an example), you can eliminate the bottle-neck where any one amino acid is concerned.

Ultimately, you can get all of your protein needs even from a strict vegan diet, so if you do not eliminate animal protein altogether, you should perhaps try to cut back on it.

Dairy products

There is conflicting information on whether dairy products can increase your risk of cancer. Research indicates that increasing your intake of calcium (and dairy products are good source of calcium) can help you to reduce your risk of bowel cancer.

However, other research indicates that there could be a link between dairy intake and the risk of developing prostate, ovarian, testicular and breast cancers because of the hormonal factors.

In Harvard's Physicians Health Study, over 20,000 male physicians were studied. They determined that those individuals who consumed two dairy servings daily (or greater), had a 34% greater risk of developing prostate cancer.

Because numerous mechanisms are involved, it is difficult to determine the root of the issue. For example, although the body requires calcium, an excessive calcium load could result in the lowering of blood levels of activated vitamin D. Vitamin D is believed to be protective against prostate cancer, so is the calcium the issue, or is it the dairy?

One other factor that gains attention from researchers is the fact that dairy product consumption increases your body's levels of IGF-1 in the bloodstream (insulin-like growth factor 1), which is a potent stimulus for the growth of cancer cells. Elevated IGF-1 levels have been linked to an increase in risk of both prostate cancer and breast cancer.

In the case of ovarian cancer, a component of the milk sugar lactose, called galactose, could be a factor. The collective analysis of a range of studies discovered that for every daily 10g of lactose consumed within dairy products, risk of ovarian cancer increased by 13%. 10g of lactose is the equivalent of one glass of milk.

In Asian countries, where vegetable sources and whole grains are commonly consumed, and milk is a much less common dietary component, the incidence of both breast cancer and prostate cancer are much lower.

Research from Harvard University has indicated perhaps the most likely factor in milk to cause cancer. It is linked to intensive factory farms in the US. It appears that high-volume, mass produced pasteurised milk from factory farms contains significantly higher levels of an oestrogen compound called estrone sulphate. In fact, up to 33 times more than grass fed cows only milked for six months after they've given birth. Factory farms often milk their cows 300 times per year, even while they are pregnant, with many being fed GMO feeds and not fresh grass.

Estrone sulphate has been shown to cause a number of hormonally driven cancers, including testicular, prostate and breast cancers.

Having evaluated data from all over the world, the Harvard researchers discovered a clear link between the consumption of this high-hormone milk and elevated rates of hormone-dependent cancers. The researchers also discovered that raw, grass fed organic milk from cows milked at appropriate times help to improve digestion, boosted immunity and reduced the impact of autoimmune disorders. So just like processed battery hen's eggs, processed battery cow milk is inferior to free range organic, and in fact could be downright dangerous.

Given the fact that, particularly in the US, cattle is also subjected to hormone injections, antibiotics, genetically modified feed, and a whole host of other unnatural processes, I would tend to limit dairy intake to fermented cheeses such as feta cheese (goats cheese), and yoghurt (without artificial sweeteners). The processes used in manufacturing these products minimise the likelihood of hormones remaining intact within the food. Failing that, opt for blue cheeses or mature versions, such as mature cheddar.

Fermented cheeses such as feta, have also been shown to be an excellent source of vitamin K2, which has demonstrated excellent cancer fighting properties in studies. Please see the Cheese section.

For milk, I prefer to use almond milk or coconut milk, which has been shown to reduce cholesterol, reduce abdominal fat and lower your risk of heart disease and type II diabetes. Equally, there is no lactose, which could be a risk factor. If you are using your milk in tea or coffee, soymilk and almond milk have less of an impact on the taste.

To ensure you are still getting enough calcium, dark green leafy vegetables, broccoli, bok choy, kale, almonds, figs, beans, mustard greens and soymilk all contain good levels of calcium, along with other additional cancer fighting nutrients. In fact, gram for gram, broccoli contains more calcium than milk.

Genetically Modified Foods (GMOs)

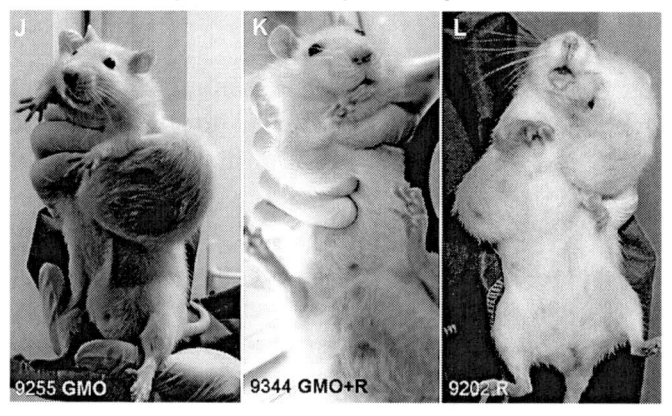

A recent peer-reviewed study (published in the Food and Chemical Toxicology Journal) has linked genetically modified foods to an increase in cancer risk in laboratory animals. In the study, the rats fed on genetically modified corn died prematurely, many of which having tumours the size of golf balls. 50% of the males and 70% of the females died prematurely as a result of a GMO diet. Not only did these rats have tumours, they also had damage to multiple organs including their liver and kidneys.

The rats were fed a form of genetically modified corn, engineered by a company called Monsanto, to resist a herbicide that they also sell, called Roundup.

This is the same type of corn often found in your corn-based breakfast cereal, corn tortillas and corn snack chips.

GMO stands for genetically modified organism. Genetically modified foods come from plants that have been genetically manipulated to exhibit different traits, including resistance to pests, resistance to weedkiller, tolerance to different temperatures and to modify the product that comes from them.

The purpose of the GMO corn being studied, was that farmers can spray their fields with the herbicide Roundup as much as they want, without killing the corn. However, Roundup has not only been linked to DNA damage and infertility, but the researchers found that Roundup-ready corn also had similar issues.

Molecular biologist, Dr. Michael Antoniou of King's College London School of Medicine explained that even the scientists involved in the study were shocked by the aggressive tumor development:

"This research shows an extraordinary number of tumors developing earlier and more aggressively – particularly in female animals. I am shocked by the extreme negative health impacts".

The danger lies in the fact that you cannot genetically manipulate one factor without triggering a raft of other changes that you did not account for. Even minor changes can have subtle effects that could be expressed over decades, as opposed to months.

In previous studies, genetically modified potatoes engineered by Monsanto were also found to have similar effects.

Jeffery Smith, author and the Executive Director of the Institute for Responsible Technology revealed:

"In the mid-90s, the UK government funded research for a scientist to figure out how to test for the safety of GMO's. That scientist was Dr Arpad Pusztai - the world's leading expert in his field. He worked at the top research laboratory in the UK. One of the best in the world. He had about 20 or 30 researchers working with him, in three different institutes. The protocols that he was designing were supposed to be implemented into EU law as requirements for the safety assessments of any GMO to be introduced into Europe.

He took a potato that was genetically engineered to produce an insecticide and fed it to one group of rats. He fed another group of rats natural potatoes and a third group of rats, natural potatoes plus their meals were spiked with the same insecticide that the modified potato was engineered to produce. So you have GM potato, natural organic potato, and natural potato plus an insecticide and all three [groups of rats] had a completely balanced diet as well.

Only the rats that ate the GM potato got sick. They had potentially precancerous cell growth in their digestive tract, smaller brains, livers and testicles, partial atrophy of the liver and damaged immune systems in 10 days. What was the cause of that damage? It was not the insecticide, because the group eating the insecticide did not have those problems. It was understood that it was the process of genetic engineering itself and the unpredicted side-effects that caused this profound damage to every system and organ studied."

According to Dr Arpad Pusztai - "Genetically Modified Foods: Potential Human Health Effects." (2003)

"We measured all sorts of things, growth for example. How these young animals were growing. What happened to their insides and what happened to their immune system and it became clear that the GM group had a slower growth. It had problems with internal development of its organs and it certainly knocked out the immune system".

"Judging by the absence of published data in peer-reviewed scientific literature, apparently no human clinical trials with GM food have ever been conducted."

"From the results, the conclusion seems inescapable that the present crude method of genetic modification has not delivered GM crops that are predictably safe and wholesome."

According to Dr Rima E. Laibow, M.D, the Medical Director of Natural Solutions Foundation, "every single independent study conducted on the impact of genetically modified food shows that it damages organs, it causes infertility, it causes immune system failure, it causes holes in the gastrointestinal tract, it causes multiple organ system failure when it is eaten. It causes a variety of changes, some of which we cannot even guess at, as new proteins are coded for by the altered DNA. [Changes] that we have never seen before. We are playing with genetic fire".

"The FDA is composed of smart people. But they are smart people with a conflict-of-interest. They are smart people who make their decisions based upon what will support their financial needs or their academic needs not what makes scientific sense."

Surprisingly, the amount of safety testing necessary to bring the product to market after genetic modification is slim to none. In fact, no human studies were required at all, and the study data Monsanto supplied involved less than 40 rats tested over just 90 days!

You may find it disturbing to discover that the FDA doesn't have a mandatory GM food safety assessment process, and as a result has never approved a genetically modified food as being safe.

Any GM food crops that have hit the commercial market so far, have only participated in a voluntary program whereby the FDA carry out a pre-market review of the GM food, based upon the data that the manufacturer presents. But this is not a legal requirement, and any research data does not have to be peer-reviewed or published.

In the US, developers of GM crops are legally allowed to put any GMO on the market, on the understanding that they can be held responsible for any harm to consumers that may result from it.

Many people do not realise the extent to which they are exposed to GMOs, nor how significantly altered these organisms are. For example, wheat in the 1950s and 60s only had 12 chromosomes in its DNA, whereas now, certain strains of wheat have 42! Humans only have 46.

In the US, the vast majority of animal feed is now genetically modified, and even in the case of GMOs for human consumption, US legislation does not require genetically modified ingredients to be labelled as such.

As of 2010, genetically modified soybeans make up 93 to 95% of the US soybean supply.

Genetically modified corn makes up 86% of the US corn supply.

Genetically modified cotton makes up 93% of the US cotton supply.

There are over 170 million acres of genetically modified crops within United States because they don't currently have to be labelled as such. These crops include maize/corn, soy beans, cotton, canola oil, sugar beets, rice, potatoes, peas and more.

In more than 50 other countries, including the UK, labelling genetically modified foods is compulsory. However, they do not have to declare if food is from animals fed GM feed, such as meat, milk or eggs.

To be on the safe side, if you notice the letters "GM", or "GMM" on your food labelling, do not eat it.

Even if you do not support the view that genetically modified crops are dangerous, you must consider the fact that the genetically modified plants are grown in environments where it is standard practice to use high levels of pesticides, which inevitably contaminate the plant itself.

According to Shiv Chopra Ph.D. "These pesticides may have killed the weeds or the insects, but the product is still on the plant. Even if it is washed off, it is still within the water supply. These compounds are toxic, they cause cancer, they cause endocryne disruption which affects your hormone levels."

So where are all the regulatory bodies who should be evaluating or putting a stop to it?

The FDA have stated that genetically engineered foods are substantially equivalent to non-genetically engineered foods. But as with the aspartame-related conflicts of interest, there are equally incestuous links between the FDA and Monsanto.

Take Michael Taylor for instance. As of 2010, he is the current deputy commissioner for foods at the FDA. Let's take a look at his career history:

1976 - Attorney for FDA
1981 - Attorney for Monsanto
1991 - Deputy Commissioner for Policy, FDA.
1998 - Vice President for Public Policy, Monsanto.
2009 - Senior Adviser to FDA Commissioner.
2010 - Deputy Commissioner for Foods, FDA.

So Monsanto's former attorney, Michael Taylor, was in charge of policy at the FDA when the GMO policy was created. He then became Monsanto's Vice President. Under the Obama administration, he was put back in the FDA as the "US food safety Tsar".

According to Joel Bakan, LL.M, Professor of Law, University of British Columbia, Film Director of "The Corporation.":

"If you look at the Clinton administration, Bush senior, Bush Jr, and Obama [administrations], you look at various high-ranking positions in the administrations of all of those presidents, you find people who've worked for Monsanto."

In the words of Jeffery Smith, author and the Executive Director of the Institute for Responsible Technology:

"In reality, the overwhelming consensus among the scientists at the FDA were not only that GMO's were different, but they were inherently dangerous. That they might create allergies, toxins, new diseases and nutritional problems. They had urged their superiors to require long-term study and when they saw drafts of the policy coming back to them, they were angry and urged their political appointees to change course. But Michael Taylor and his local appointees ignored the science, ignored the scientists, denied the existence of their concerns and set forth a policy that allowed GMO's to be put on the market in a way that creates unprecedented risk for human beings and the environment."

"Monsanto originally said that PCBs were safe. They were [subsequently] convicted of actually poisoning the people in the town next to the PCB factory and were fined $700 million. They told us that agent Orange was safe, they told us that DDT was safe and now they are in charge of telling us whether their own genetically modified foods are safe because the FDA does not require a single safety study. They leave it to Monsanto."

"When genetically modified soy beans were fed to rodents, we have seen changes in the testicles, changes in the sperm cells, changes in uterus and overies, in the DNA functioning of the embryo offspring, smaller babies with a death rate that is 5 times higher compared with controls. Sterile babies, even babies born with hair in their mouths.

This research has been done by government scientists, and scientists who were at the top of their field."

So can you trust Monsanto? Phil Angell, Monsanto's Director of Corporate Communications, quoted in the New York Times, October 25, 1998 said:

"Monsanto should not have to vouchsafe the safety of biotech food. Our interest is in selling as much of it as possible. Assuring safety is the FDA's job."

Both France and Russia have recently banned GMO crops, so we shall soon see if other countries follow suit.

Regardless of what your government decides, in the interests of remaining cancer free, and maximising your health, you should personally avoid genetically modified ingredients in your foods.

Hydrogenated fats and trans fats

Trans-fat is only found in trace amounts in some natural foods. However, with today's modern food manufacturing and processing, large quantities of these dangerous fatty acids are formed when vegetable oil is processed, especially during hydrogenation. Hydrogenation is used to prolong shelflife and to initiate the texture of certain saturated fats, such as margarine.

A 2008 study, conducted by the University of North Carolina and published in the American Journal of Epidemiology, showed that people who consume the highest levels of trans fat increased their risk of colon cancer by 86%. This is as significant to colon cancer as cigarette smoking is to lung cancer.

They found that the more trans fat somebody consumes, the more precancerous polyps are found in their colon. They defined the higher levels of consumption of trans fat being an average of 6.5g per day.

Previous research has linked trans fat to increased risk of heart disease, infertility, breast cancer and now colon cancer.

To avoid trans fats, you cannot simply rely on product claims of having no trans fats. You must check the label, because sometimes on the ingredients list you will still find hydrogenated oil, which can give you up to half a gram of trans fat per serving.

Due to labelling regulations, if the food contains anything less than 0.49 g of trans fat per serving, it can be listed as 0g on the "Nutritional Facts" section.

Some of the many foods that contain trans fat include:

French fries and almost anything else deep-fried or battered, pies and piecrust, certain brands of margarine, certain cake mixes and frostings, pancakes and waffle mixes, fried chicken, certain nondairy creamers, ground beef, beef hotdogs, frozen burgers, cookies, biscuits, certain breakfast cereals, certain chewy granola bars, Special K cereal bars, Girl Scout cookies, crisps/potato chips, certain brands of popcorn, Animal Crackers, Ritz Crackers, Fortune cookies, restaurant milkshakes (a 20 ounce Chocolate Chip Cookie Dough Arctic Avalanche provided by Krispy Kreme, contains a whopping 9g of trans fats in one serving!), Frozen dinners and microwave meals, canned Chili, and more.

Acrylamide

Acrylamide is a known neurotoxin and carcinogen that is formed in certain foods when they are fried or baked at high temperatures. Foods high in carbohydrates and/or an amino acid called asparagine are particularly susceptable.

In laboratory tests, commissioned by the Centre for Science in the Public Interest (CSPI) in 2002, researchers discovered alarming levels in some commercially available foods.

For example, the amount of acrylamide in a large order of fast-food French fries was at least 300 times more than what the U.S. Environmental Protection Agency allows in a glass of water. Acrylamide is sometimes used in water-treatment facilities.

Based upon standard EPA projections of risk from animal studies, research professor Dale Hattis of Clark University warned "I estimate that acrylamide causes several thousand cancers per year in Americans."

Here are some of the test results:

Acrylamide in Foods:	Micrograms per Serving
Water, 8 oz. (EPA limit)	0.12
Old El Paso Taco Shells, 3, 1.1oz.	1
Boiled Potatoes, 4 oz.	<3
Ore Ida French Fries (uncooked), 3 oz	5

Tostitos Tortilla Chips, 1 oz.	5
Honey Nut Cheerios, 1 oz.	6
Cheerios, 1 oz.	7
Fritos Corn Chips, 1 oz.	11
Pringles Potato Crisps, 1 oz.	25
Ore Ida French Fries (baked), 3 oz.	28
Wendy's French Fries, Biggie, 5.6 oz.	39
KFC Potato Wedges, Jumbo, 6.2 oz.	52
Burger King French Fries, large, 5.7 oz.	59
McDonald's French Fries, large, 6.2 oz.	82

While scientists do not know for sure, it is believed that avoiding the cooking and re-cooking of fried foods in a previously used and unwashed pan, should reduce your exposure. Equally, this data indicates that it would be wise to avoid foods that are deep fried by restaurants which use the same oil over and over.

In 2006, the United States Food and Drug Administration released the results of its most recent research on the acrylamide content of common foods.

The top 20 foods by average acrylamide intake by the U.S. population are as follows:

1. French Fries (made in restaurants)
2. French Fries (oven baked)
3. Potato Chips
4. Breakfast Cereals
5. Cookies
6. Brewed Coffee
7. Toast
8. Pies and Cakes
9. Crackers
10. Soft Bread
11. Chili con Carne
12. Corn Snacks

13. Popcorn
14. Pretzels
15. Pizza
16. Burrito/Tostada
17. Peanut Butter
18. Breaded Chicken
19. Bagels
20. Soup Mix

Monosodium glutamate

Monosodium glutamate, otherwise known as MSG, is a controversial food additive designed to enhance flavour.

There are two kinds of MSG. Natural MSG, otherwise known as L-glutamic acid, is derived from a range of plant and animal-based foods found in the diet of most people. It is a harmless amino acid when it is bound with proteins, which allows your body to absorb it slowly and naturally. Manufactured and processed MSG is another story.

Man-made MSG is free glutamic acid, which does not have any protein component to slow down its absorption, which is then mixed with salt. After salt-and-pepper, MSG is now the third most common flavour enhancer. It works by tricking your brain into believing the food you eat tastes good, and this is used by the food industry to make substandard ingredients taste better.

The danger lies in the fact that glutamate is also used as part of your central nervous system as a neurotransmitter in the brain. It helps to regulate the central nervous system and is required for normal brain and organ function. Glutamate is believed to play a role in memory and learning.

By consuming man-made MSG, we are able to flood our bodies with glutamate, which, whilst triggering a "better" taste in our food, also risks interfering with our natural neurological processes.

A spike of MSG can overstimulate brain neurons, leading to both physical and psychological problems. Some people are more sensitive to the effects than others, due to their age, levels of stress or perhaps existing disease, but symptoms of too much MSG include migraines, an asthma attack, stuffy nose, throat swelling, diarrhoea, skin rash, irregular heartbeats or even the mimic of a stroke or heart attack. Tests have shown that a high enough dose of MSG can make **everyone** experience an immediate reaction.

Long-term exposure of MSG has been implicated in a wide range of conditions (including cancer), such as mood swings, depression, infertility, paranoia, Parkinson's disease, Alzheimer's disease, memory loss, obesity, birth defects, retinal damage, learning disabilities and more.

Animal studies in 2006 showed that MSG damages blood vessels, through the action of free radicals, which can lead to weakened arteries and blood clots.

With regard to cancer, the primary concern is that many cancers have been shown to have glutamate receptors. MSG is able to bind to these glutamate receptors, stimulating the growth of the cancer cells.

A paper published in Oxford Journals / International Immunology showed that cancer patients typically have high glutamate levels. They also showed that lung cancer patients with the lowest glutamate levels had the highest survival rates. High glutamate levels also appear to reduce your cells' ability to absorb another amino acid called cystine.

Cystine is used to make glutathione as well as taurine, which are naturally occurring water-soluble antioxidants that help to detoxify your cells and protect against the damage caused by free radicals.

Glutathione has shown to have excellent anti-cancer properties both in terms of prevention and inhibiting cancer cell growth. Excellent sources of glutathione include asparagus, Brazil nuts and whey protein. Glutathione is also contained in potatoes, carrots, onions, avocados, spinach, tomatoes, broccoli, peppers, oranges, apples, bananas and grapefruit.

Your body also needs selenium in order to form glutathione containing enzymes, so consumption of Brazil nuts, walnuts, cheese, eggs, poultry, beef and tuna may be beneficial for this reason.

The general consensus of the Oxford Journals' published research is that reducing your glutamate levels should increase your body's cancer fighting ability.

Supporting this, a study published by the National Academy of Sciences showed that glutamate antagonists (which counteract glutamate) limited the tumour growth in colon cancer, breast cancer, brain cancer and lung cancer cells. Glutamate antagonists also decreased the motility and invasive growth of tumour cells.

In addition, not only can the glutamate itself cause a problem, but two out of the five types of MSG manufacturing process also create low levels of carcinogenic impurities. Manufacturing MSG via acid hydrolysis creates small amounts of carcinogenic mono and dichloro propanols and MSG produced via a Maillard reaction, always contains traces of carcinogenic heterocyclic amines. Heterocyclic amines are the same carcinogens you get in charred or burnt food.

Despite MSG being classified by the FDA as "GRAS", (generally recognised as safe), the FDA persistently receive complaints of negative side-effects from this product.

Worse still, if you want to cut this additive out of your diet, food manufacturers have become increasingly crafty about how they label it. If it isn't labelled as MSG or monosodium glutamate, it may be disguised as textured protein, sodium caseinate, hydrolysed vegetable protein and soy protein isolate. Sometimes, it may not even be listed. For example when it is added to some raw fruits and vegetables in the preservative wax coating.

The only way to truly avoid it altogether, is to prepare your own foods from fresh ingredients. Anyone considering avoiding monosodium glutamate should also avoid aspartame, because it breaks down into glutamate, phenylalanine and methanol.

Preservatives, including phosphates

Whilst we have already discussed the negative impact of nitrites in cured and processed meats, research published in the 2009 issue of the American Journal of Respiratory and Critical Care Medicine highlighted the dangers of processed foods containing inorganic phosphates.

Inorganic phosphates are used as an additive to increase water retention, and to improve the texture of certain processed foods.

In many countries, food manufacturers are not required to list phosphate levels on the "Nutritional Facts" part of the label. In fact, they are often not required to monitor phosphate levels at all.

Prior research has shown links between inorganic phosphate consumption and the premature ageing of tissues, chronic kidney disease, weak bones and premature death. But beyond this, research conducted by the American Thoracic Society, showed that diets high in inorganic phosphates may also significantly increase your risk of lung cancer.

Concerns relating to the impact of the phosphate content in processed foods on human health have been raised in the European medical Journal (Deutsches Ärzteblatt International), which called for stronger labelling laws requiring phosphate content to be listed.

In the 2009 study, lung cancer-model mice were studied over a four-week period, having been randomly assigned a diet of either 0.5% or 1% phosphate, which is in the range of modern diets. At the conclusion of the four-week study, the effects of the inorganic phosphates were determined by analysing the lung tissue.

The results clearly demonstrated that the higher the concentration of inorganic phosphates, the greater the size of the tumours found. The study indicated that inorganic phosphates strongly stimulate lung cancer development in mice, and should therefore be avoided in order to increase the success rate of lung cancer treatment and as part of a lung cancer prevention strategy in healthy people.

Lung cancer is currently the official number one cause of cancer-related death worldwide (if you discount our own doctors and harmful / ineffective treatments), so trying to avoid sources of inorganic phosphates is certainly a good idea.

Sources of inorganic phosphates are currently hard to spot, due to the lax labelling requirements. In fact, there are over 45 different phosphate related additives in processed foods. Look out for "sodium phosphate", "calcium phosphate", "phosphoric acid", and numerous other variations.

It is true that we need phosphorus to survive, but naturally occurring phosphorus found in eggs, meat, fish, poultry, nuts, whole grains, legumes and dairy products is organic phosphorus and our body can only absorb around 40 to 60% of it. Unfortunately, inorganic phosphate additives are much more readily absorbed, meaning that we can end up with excessive levels of phosphate within our blood.

We are only supposed to have around 700mg per day of phosphorus, and yet many people unwittingly consume in excess of 1500mg.

The worst culprits for inorganic phosphate additives are frozen dinners, baked goods, processed meats, convenience foods (such as flavoured noodles), some sodas, fast foods and restaurant foods in general, and unfortunately, some calcium fortified foods that are fortified with calcium phosphate.

Keep an eye out for anything on food labels beginning "phos-", and preferably avoid it.

Pickled foods

Pickled foods can lead to an increase in stomach and oesophageal cancer risk. In fact, the World Health Organisation has listed pickled vegetables as a possible carcinogen.

A recent study, published in the British Journal of Cancer 2009, concluded that data obtained from 34 different studies showed a two-fold increase in the risk of oesophageal cancer in those who consume pickled vegetables on a regular basis.

Intermittent use of pickled vegetables, such as gherkins, is not likely to cause significant increases in risk. But some of the studies were conducted on people in parts of China where pickled vegetables were eaten daily for between 9 and 12 months of the year, and these showed an undeniable connection.

By the same token, there is also a correlation between bulimia and an increased risk of oesophageal cancer, perhaps because the persistent action of acid on the oesophagus is not good for the squamous cells, which line the oesophagus.

Refined sugar and sugar alcohols

Whilst I would advocate refined sugar over artificial sweeteners, excess blood sugar levels are known to age almost every tissue in your body. High blood sugar also puts a load on your pancreas, which is forced to produce ever-increasing amounts of insulin in order to get your fat cells to store up the excess sugar, before it causes damage to your brain, eyes and other tissues.

The biggest risks from excess sugar include diabetes, obesity, heart disease and cancer. Many people do not realise that the direct cause of high cholesterol in your bloodstream is actually your body trying to process and store the excess sugar. If you have high cholesterol, you need to consider how much sugar and carbohydrates are in your diet.

Whilst it is fairly straightforward to limit table sugar, (which you may add to hot drinks and breakfast cereals), many of the sources of sugar are not readily identifiable, even from food labelling.

For example, high fructose corn syrup (derived from highly processed corn), doesn't necessarily sound like sugar.

Table sugar, otherwise known as sucrose, is derived from sugar beets or sugar cane. Fructose, is derived from fruits, lactose comes from milk, and maltose comes from malted foods, including barley.

Perhaps the easiest way to moderate your sugar intake is to pay attention to the glycaemic index of foods.

Glycaemic index (GI) is a measure of how significantly a food will influence your blood sugar levels, and how quickly it does it. This number ranges from 1 to 100, with pure glucose (blood sugar) being set at 100.

A low glycaemic index, say from 1 to 40, means that the food will have a release of energy that will not dramatically influence your blood sugar levels. For example, olives or a piece of cheese will make little or no difference to your blood sugar levels.

However, medium (50 to 70) or high (70 and above) glycaemic index foods will have a more dramatic impact.

Glycaemic index is important because if you persistently get surges of blood sugar, you are overtaxing your blood sugar stabilising mechanisms (which can lead to diabetes). The secondary effect, is that after you have released a load of insulin to help store the sugar, you get a blood sugar dip. This low blood sugar level triggers a mechanism in the brain related to cravings. On that basis, high sugar foods can give your body a boom and bust cycle of blood sugar, which generally results in your consuming more calories and putting on weight.

Most fruit and vegetables have a low glycaemic index, with the exception of potatoes and bananas, which have a medium glycaemic index. This means that you can eat fruit and vegetables without causing undue load on your hormone systems and waistline. This is an all-round healthier option.

As soon as you start looking at the man-made and processed food options, such as pretzels, white bread, and anything containing high fructose corn syrup, you are in the realms of a high glycaemic index.

When considering your sources of sugar, you must realise that not all sugars are created equal. Gram for gram, even if they contain the same amount of calories, their glycaemic index can be quite different because of the way they are processed in the body:

Stevia 0
Xylitol 7
Agave Nectar 15-30
Fructose 17
Brown Rice Syrup 25
Raw Honey 30
Organic Sugar 47
Turbinado 65
Raw Sugar 65
Cola 70
Corn Syrup 75
Table Sugar 80
High Fructose Corn Syrup 87

Glucose/Dextrose 100

So what should you avoid? A study conducted by Princeton University demonstrated that rats gained significantly more weight when consuming high fructose corn syrup (HFCS) compared with rats consuming table sugar (sucrose) even when the total caloric intake was identical. In fact, the rats consuming HFCS gained 48% more weight and had noticeable deposits of abdominal fat and elevated levels of triglycerides in their bloodstream. Translated into human terms, this would basically indicate obesity, with a high risk of heart disease, diabetes and cancer.

In an effort to go under the radar of more health-conscious consumers, high fructose corn syrup is now sometimes renamed corn sugar.

But it isn't just about excesses of sugar causing strain on your endocrine system. Different sugars are broken down differently, and some can put more strain on your body (and use more resources) than others.

Glucose can travel straight into the bloodstream and be utilised by every single cell in the body. Fructose, however, has to be processed in the liver before the body can use it. In fruit, the sugar ratio is typically 50% glucose and 50% fructose, but the absorption of the fructose is slowed down by the presence of fibre within the fruit. This means that although you are making your liver work, it is done at a sustained and manageable rate. The enzymes and vitamins necessary to process the fruit sugar are mainly provided within the fruit itself.

High fructose corn syrup can be manipulated to the degree where it is 80% fructose and only 20% glucose, with lots of "free fructose". The fructose is not bound to other sugars, slowed down by the fruit fibre, nor supplemented with the necessary vitamins and minerals. As a result, high fructose corn syrup can tax your liver and rob your body of its vitamin and mineral reserves.

The US Department of agriculture investigated the effect on rats of high levels of fructose. They discovered that when rats were fed a high fructose diet, which was simultaneously deficient in copper, the rats developed organ problems. Their livers, hearts and testes exhibited extreme swelling, whilst their pancreases atrophied, which invariably led to their deaths before maturity.

When rats were put in the same situation, except with glucose as the main carbohydrate source, the rats showed some sign of copper deficiency, but did not have the major organ abnormalities.

Studies have shown that higher fructose diets result in mineral losses, with especially high faecal excretion of iron and magnesium, and greater urinary excretion of magnesium and phosphorus.

High levels of fructose ingestion in people also increases the amount of lactic acid in the blood, which may have further implications. It has been shown that cancer cells thrive in an acidic environment.

Elevated fructose levels can also interfere with copper metabolism. Modern diets are relatively low in copper anyway, so adding high fructose corn syrup into the equation can further exacerbate the problem. Copper deficiency can lead to anaemia, bone fragility, tissue defects, heart arrhythmias, heart attacks, high cholesterol levels and even infertility.

High fructose corn syrup is the primary sweetener used in soft drinks. This is particularly worrying when some of the greatest consumers are our children. In the US, soft drink consumption among children has virtually doubled in the last 10 years. In fact, teenage boys drink on average three or more cans of soft drinks per day. 10% of them drink upwards of seven cans per day.

When it comes to commercially available food, the best thing you can do is to read the label and look for foods that do not contain high fructose corn syrup. Equally, choose foods that are known to be of a medium or low glycaemic index. The best option is to consume your food as close to raw as possible, which often means natural produce, without the addition of sugar.

If you do have to use a sweetener, then Honey is a great choice, not only because of its low glycaemic index, but also because of the enzymes and naturally occurring nutrients within it.

Sugar alcohols are another form of artificial sweetener. They are basically a hydrogenated form of carbohydrate which is often used in commercial foods, and are known as polyol, polyhydric alcohol, Polyalcohol or glycitol.

The most common sugar alcohols include arabitol, mannitol, maltitol, xylitol and sorbitol, and are sometimes labelled as hydrogenated starch hydrolysates.

There are several advantages of using sugar alcohols for the food manufacturers, but considerably less advantages for the consumer.

Firstly, because these substances aren't technically sugar (although part of their chemical structure resembles sugar), they do not have to be listed as sugar on the ingredients label. As a result, they are frequently used in "sugar-free" foods.

The label of "sugar-free" is not the same as carbohydrate-free or calorie-free, but this distinction is often not understood, and lures consumers in with the impression of consequence-free snacking.

The fact of the matter is that sugar alcohols do still moderately affect your blood sugar levels, even if they are not listed as being sugar. Equally, they are typically used in carbohydrate-rich foods which may well have a fairly high glycaemic index.

Secondly, whilst you can detect the sweetness of sugar alcohols, (around 60-80% as sweet as sucrose), in many cases their absorption is quite poor. So food manufacturers can use quite a lot of them without it adding greatly to the calorie count. This might sound like a good idea, but whilst your body may have difficulty absorbing and utilising the sugar alcohols, the bacteria in your gut does not.

As a result, excessive consumption of sugar alcohols can lead to a laxative effect as they ferment in the gut, giving symptoms including flatulence, diarrhoea, and bloating. This is worse in people susceptible to irritable bowel syndrome.

Thirdly, they are often used to disguise the unpleasant aftertaste of other, more potent, artificial sweeteners and are used to improve the taste of nutritionally-dead junk food.

The only real advantage to the consumer is that sugar alcohols are not typically broken down and fermented by oral bacteria, which means that sugar-free gum manufacturers can sweeten their product without causing dental cavities.

In conclusion, whilst sugar alcohol itself hasn't been shown to cause a great deal of harm, beyond abdominal discomfort, the kind of foods they are typically put into are not the healthy, nutritious, enzyme-rich fresh foods that you should be aiming for in order to reduce your risk of cancer.

Very hot tea

As bizarre as this sounds, studies have been conducted that demonstrate that people who regularly drink their tea at temperatures exceeding 70°C have a significantly higher risk of oesophageal cancer.

Primary causes of oesophageal cancer are smoking and the consumption of alcohol, but the British medical Journal highlighted the evidence from this study as an additional factor.

Wheat

As I mentioned in the Genetically Modified Foods section, commercial wheat is a completely different plant than it was just 50 or 60 years ago.

A book that I would heartily recommend, is "Wheat belly", by William Davis MD. It details the fact that wheat has been grossly manipulated (over the course of decades) into a new and potentially dangerous product.

It has gone from a 12 chromosome grass to a 42 chromosome abomination that, as Dr Davis points out, exaggerates blood sugar levels, triggers allergic reactions, triggers cycles of alternating satiety and hunger, damages a wide range of tissues through glycation, causes inflammatory effects and influences your body pH (thereby eroding cartilage, bone and fostering an acidic environment) and activates a disordered immune response.

The very name "Wheat Belly" comes from the fact that the persistent insulin response caused by wheat consumption triggers a buildup of visceral fat (fat around your middle), as this is the emergency dumping ground for fat.

Abdominal fat is the greatest indicator of risk for heart disease and diabetes, and it correlates with a high consumption of wheat. Worse than that, visceral fat has a habit of provoking inflammatory responses, it can distort insulin responses and can produce oestrogen in both women and men, potentially creating "man breasts" or an increased risk of breast cancer.

Research published in the Journal of the National Cancer Institute showed that postmenopausal women with high levels of visceral fat can have up to a four-fold increase in the risk of breast cancer.

As Dr Davis says, "the consequences of wheat consumption, however, are not just manifested on the body's surface; wheat can also reach deep down into virtually every organ of the body, from the intestines, liver, heart, and thyroid gland all the way up to the brain. In fact, there is hardly an organ that is not affected by wheat in some potentially damaging way."

Dr Davis is a cardiologist, so as part of his day-to-day interaction with patients, he was focused upon helping them to reduce their body weight, lower cholesterol levels and improve their general health.

He noticed a dramatic contrast between the healthy and slender individuals of the 1950s and the overweight, prediabetic, tired and run-down people of today.

Looking at the symptoms his patients were experiencing, alongside the dramatic increase in coeliac disease, gluten intolerance, and allergies over the last 50 years, Dr Davis realised that one of the common factors linking everything together, was the systematic modification of one of the staples of the Western diet. Wheat.

A range of changes have been instigated in wheat over the years, in order to increase its yield, change its resistance to pests, improve its resistance to climates and weather conditions, alter the texture and properties of its flour, and more. For example, wheat is now 2 feet shorter, and the structure of the carbohydrate within it is now different, making it much more easily absorbed.

In fact, a slice of wholemeal bread (with its easily digestible carbohydrate, amylopectin A) has a higher (worse) glycaemic index and gives you a bigger blood sugar spike than 6 teaspoons of table sugar. It is worse for a diabetic than giving them a candy bar!

With every new strain of hybrid plant, (whether from selective breeding or from genetic modification), the possibility of unanticipated proteins being coded for in the DNA increases exponentially. As a result, in addition to gluten (which may trigger allergy or intolerances), wheat also contains an appetite-stimulating protein called gliadin.

A study in the Journal of Biological Chemistry, showed that when the proteins in wheat are broken down with hydrochloric acid and digestive enzymes, (simulating digestion) the resulting mix of polypeptides were found to contain morphine-like compounds able to cross the blood-brain barrier in rats, binding to the opiate receptors in their brains. The exact same receptors that heroin would bind to.

The researchers called these opiate-like compounds "exorphins", which was short for exogenous morphine-like compounds, (as opposed to endorphins, which are endogenous morphine-like compounds, that your body generates during exercise to make you feel good). The most common variant was named "gluteomorphin".

Scientists have since discovered that when rats are administered naloxone, a drug used to block the effect of heroin, it also blocks the effects of wheat exorphins.

This chemical reward, triggered by consuming wheat, is likely to induce a mild euphoria and could potentially make wheat addictive. If you were cynical, you might wonder if the multibillion-dollar a year wheat industry engineered this in on purpose?

The gliadin and exorphin combination is certainly very effective in promoting the repeat consumption of wheat. On average, those who consume wheat in their diet have a daily calorie intake 460 calories higher than those who don't.

Dr Davis' research led him to discover the ample scientific studies illustrating the negative impact of modern wheat, so after following his own advice, and seeing the benefits, he started to recommend a wheat-free diet to his patients.

Since then, Dr Davis reports literally thousands of his patients having dramatic improvements in health, including weight loss (30 lbs to 50 lbs within the first few months being typical), a reduction in allergies, being able to eliminate diabetes medication, the elimination of joint pain and in extreme cases, the avoidance of scheduled surgery. In many of these cases, the changes in diet, lifestyle and body weight, significantly reduced the risk of cancer.

As a direct result of this book, and the scientific insight of Dr Davis, I now happily live on a wheat-free diet. I lost 16 lbs of unwanted body fat within the first 60 days, (23lbs in the first 90 days), significantly improved my complexion and noticeably improved my levels of energy. My cravings for food disappeared after the first three days, making me less distracted and more productive.

By removing wheat from my diet, it forced me to evaluate my food choices, often opting for raw fruit and vegetables, nuts, seeds, fish, eggs, cheese and generally more nutritious options, which keep my blood sugar completely stable.

Without specifically intending to, (and without being hungry), I have reduced my daily caloric intake by approximately 500 calories, and significantly improved my nutrition. I now live the advice I offer in this book, so I know everything I recommend is achievable. Better yet, I feel fantastic. Thank you Dr Davis!

You can read more about the Wheat Belly book at:

http://www.CancerUncensored.com/wheat-belly

Looking for wheat on food labels is a great start in trying to avoid it, but the food industry has discovered that there are covert ways to label wheat products so that they go under the radar of the average consumer. Non-specific terms including "leavening agents", "starch" or "emulsifiers" should be considered sources of wheat until proven otherwise.

Having lived this lifestyle myself, I do acknowledge that living wheat-free is not easy if you have a busy schedule. After all, you can't take your kitchen with you when you go to work, or out for the day. I try to plan ahead and pack mixed nuts, fruit / dried fruit or salads with me, but if I have to eat out, then I opt for non-wheat options like curry and rice, soups, baked potatoes, salads, etc. You can usually find something to eat if you get creative!

You can read more about the impact of allergies and food intolerance in the Allergy section of this book.

Junk food

Junk food tends to be an amalgam of all of the nasty additives I have listed. Take a US corn dog for example... A collection of trans fats, nitrites, acrylamide, and inorganic phosphates, wrapped up in a potentially genetically modified, vitamin and mineral depleted corn coating, containing no enzymes to help you break it down. 0% Vitamin C, 0% vitamin A, 50% of the calories from fat. Hmmm delicious!

In junk food, if it isn't the preservatives, the refined sugar, the MSG or artificial sweeteners, excessive salt, the freakish modern "Frankenstein" wheat, or the hydrogenated fats or animal fats, then it is likely to be something else equally harmful to your health! No wonder cancer rates have increased so drastically.

They don't call it junk food for nothing. Aside from the harmful additives, it is generally devoid of nutrition. The bottom line is that if you are going to indulge, try not to do it too often.

Examples of junk food include: crisps / potato chips / corn chips, soda or soft drinks, fast food, commercial milkshakes, pizza, doughnuts, candy bars, sweets, biscuits / cookies, pork rinds / pork scratchings, and ice cream.

Why not trade in your junk food for fresh organic yoghurt with chopped fruit, or freeze-dried organic berries, or a tasty spiced fresh soup, or a delicious chicken or tuna salad with a tasty dressing?

Believe me, I used to watch diet programs on television, where they used to shock overweight people by putting all the junk they ate in a week on a table (or even sliding it down a chute into a bucket), and as shocking as it was supposed to be, it made my mouth water! I loved my junk food!

But after just a few weeks of eating fresh, I couldn't go back. Your taste buds change, your body detoxifies and you can't imagine eating nutritionally dead, yellow freezer-food. You don't change to this lifestyle and maintain it because it's good for you, it is because you can **feel** the difference, and fresh, natural produce **tastes better**... and you can eat as much of it as you want!

Try to remember, if it hasn't come straight from nature, there are probably nasty additives in there that you should avoid.

Be ruthless for the first two weeks. Stick rigidly to your diet, and the habit will kick in until it becomes second nature and effortless. I decided to commit to a 30 day trial, and by day 30, there was no way I was going back!

Anticancer Activities

In addition to eating well and avoiding foods known to increase your risk of cancer, there are a range of other factors to consider. This section covers the activities that can actively reduce your cancer risk.

Enjoy Exercise

Whilst a link between exercise and good health is fairly intuitive, many people do not realise how dramatic the link is.

A recent study conducted by researchers at Bristol University, which comprehensively reviewed over 182 prior studies, showed that regular physical activity could decrease your risk of cancer by as much as 50%.

Exercise was shown to have a significant impact upon the prevention of, and recovery from, bowel cancer, breast cancer, prostate cancer, lung cancer and even endometrial cancer.

Focusing in on studies specifically related to bowel cancer, the researchers found that regular exercise could cut the risk of developing bowel cancer by 40 to 50%.

Looking at 52 studies relating to exercise and breast cancer, they discovered that women who regularly exercised had an average 30% reduction in their breast cancer risk.

A separate review of 40 different studies, published in the International Journal of Clinical Practice 2010, spanning from 2006 to 2010 showed that aside from quitting smoking, getting more exercise was the single biggest thing somebody could do to improve their health. In fact, exercise reduced the risk of over 24 different major physical and mental conditions.

The American Cancer Association estimates that 14-20% of cancer deaths are due to obesity and that 24.2% of American adults do no exercise whatsoever. In some states it was as high as 33% of adults.

The thing with regular activity is that you should not simply look at it as a way to improve the health of your heart and lungs, it also helps your body move the fluid in your lymphatic system, which is an integral part of your immune system.

Your blood is pumped around your body by your heart, but your lymphatic system, which carries white blood cells and helps your body to detoxify, does not have its own pumping mechanism. It relies upon the movement of your muscles to push the fluid around your body.

I am sure the lymphatic system was not designed to operate effectively for somebody who sits all day at a desk, who then sits in their car on their way home, to sit in front of the TV, before lying in bed. How does this lifestyle encourage your immune system to circulate effectively, and remove the build-up of toxins from your system?

So yes, 45 min of reasonably strenuous exercise three times per week, or 30 minutes five times per week, or even 20 min per day would be great (even if it is just a brisk walk around the block), but really you should find an excuse to move around for 10 minutes every hour or so.

I no longer think of exercise as being "exercise", I think of it as a way to power up my immune system and detoxify my body by pumping my lymphatic system.

It is also a good idea to try and find activities that do not seem like exercise. Playing catch or frisbee with your kids, walking round the block hand-in-hand with your spouse after dinner, discussing your day, or using the stairs instead of the elevator, add little incremental boosts to your general health. It isn't just about heading to the gym to grind out some quality time on the treadmill. It can be as easy as doing a few squats, or sit-ups in front of your favourite TV show. Or even marching on the spot during the ad breaks. Make it a game.

Another function of exercise is that it increases your body's production of its own natural antioxidants, which decreases the impact of free radicals (that age your tissues and increase the risk of cancer). Long-term activity helps you to maintain the number of mitochondria in your cells, which normally decrease in size and number as you age.

Mitochondria are responsible for converting sugar into energy, so this age-related reduction can predispose you to gaining weight.

Keeping active therefore has the triple effect of pumping your lymphatic system, increasing your levels of antioxidants and enabling you to burn more calories while at rest, (which helps you to maintain a healthy bodyweight).

Just find reasons to move your body and it will serve you much better in the long-run. Don't even think of it as short-term improvements, but consider that in retirement, it is the difference between actively participating in life (and family), or having to watch it from your armchair or sick-bed.

Seek out moderate sun exposure

Dr Mercola, in his YouTube video "How to cut your risk of cancer in half", shares that there is a significant correlation between where you live and your risk of cancer. He shows that the further away from the equator you get, the greater your statistical cancer risk. This correlates to a reduction in the amount and intensity of sun exposure throughout the year.

This, in turn, affects your bodily levels of vitamin D. Your body converts cholesterol into vitamin D in the presence of sunlight, and vitamin D is a powerful antioxidant. On that basis, to gain the health benefits, you can either try to get greater sun exposure or else consume more vitamin D.

As Dr Mercola explains, it is far safer to gain vitamin D from sun exposure, due to the risk of overdosing your vitamin D consumption when taken orally. But do NOT get sunburn, as this increases skin cancer risk.

If you have dark skin, you get less of the vitamin D being created by sun exposure due to the fact that the melanin in your skin is screening out the UVB rays.

As I mentioned in the Fish section of this book, insufficient vitamin D levels are linked to pretty much every age-related disorder there is, including heart disease, cancer, chronic inflammation, depression, autoimmune diseases, diabetes and osteoporosis.

If you have no choice but to obtain your vitamin D from your diet, then oily fish including salmon, mackerel, tuna and sardines are an excellent source.

If you can't bring yourself to consume greater quantities of fish, then use a supplement containing vitamin D3 (cholecalciferol). Be aware however, that vitamin D2, a synthetic form of vitamin D is not the same and has not been shown to have the same anti-cancer benefits.

Get plenty of sleep

"A good laugh and a long sleep are the best cures in the doctor's book." - An Irish Proverb

Studies have shown that people who sleep for less than six hours each night have a 50% greater risk of developing polyps in the colon, which are known to lead to colon cancer. When you sleep, you produce a hormone called melatonin, which acts as an antioxidant. If you sleep for less than six hours per night, your body simply cannot produce enough to repair your cells, keeping cancer at bay.

Another study involved postmenopausal breast cancer patients. The participants in the study were all tested with Oncotype DX, which is a tool that doctors can use to predict whether breast cancer will recur. They compared this with survey data from patients about their sleep habits for the last two years. They discovered a sharp increase in the test scores for women who got less than six hours sleep per night. The researchers concluded that "the lack of sufficient sleep may cause more aggressive tumours".

It is perhaps more likely that it is not the tumour that is affected, but your body's ability to fight it with reduced melatonin levels.

Some experts suggest setting an alarm clock for your bedtime, just in the same way as you would set an alarm clock to get up in the morning. This will ensure that you get eight hours of sleep.

Colonic massage

There is a growing mass of medical data that shows that toxicity in the body often begins in the colon. Undigested, decomposing food can get backed up in our digestive tract, forming a nasty lining within our colons, that has been coined "mucosal plaque".

This buildup can distend the colon, increasing its diameter and reducing its ability to expel our waste efficiently. This then results in our livers being overworked, and our blood gradually carrying more toxins. In theory, if you clear the bowel, you can then clear the liver, which in turn, clears the blood.

Whilst there are an array of purgatives and laxatives designed to cleanse your colon, and colonic irrigation (sometimes referred to as hydrotherapy) to flush out the toxic buildup, I am also aware of the three pounds of beneficial bacteria that is common to most people's intestines. I am not entirely convinced that flooding your bowel with water is the best way to cleanse it.

This is where colonic massage fits in. During a 25 to 30 minute process, the masseur stimulates the blood flow and musculature of the colon, by circular motion on the abdomen, and the application of pressure to specific regions in a sequence.

This form of massage has been shown to remove inches from your waistline and remove significant amounts of waste material the next time you go to the toilet.

My own experience was a relatively pleasant one. The process was generally relaxing, whilst only having minor and intermittent discomfort when the deepest tissues were massaged, towards the end of the process. The immediate result, without being too graphic, was that the waste material I produced after the massage was much darker than usual, and was more loose. It certainly didn't look like something I would normally produce.

This is normally something that is repeated as a series of treatments, followed by intermittent maintenance treatments. In my case, it cost £30 for a session, which is the equivalent of just under $50 US.

The longer-term result has been an increase in the frequency of using the bathroom, which indicates an improvement in function. An improvement in diet has no doubt had a positive impact, so it is difficult to determine where to attribute the improvements.

Certainly there has been an entire turnaround in the consistency of the material, which I am glad to report is a vast improvement. So whilst visits to the bathroom are more frequent, they take moments and involve minimal fuss.

A supplement that I added to my diet recently, (and which I now could not imagine being without), is called "SuperGreens" and is manufactured by Living Fuel Inc. It is a natural-source meal replacement powder, which includes natural plant fibre, complete protein from vegetable sources, antioxidants, vitamins and minerals, essential fatty acids, probiotics and enzymes. One complete serving (2 scoops) contains the equivalent of 12 portions of fruit and vegetables!

Even just consuming half of 1 serving per day, (thereby using it as a supplement instead of a meal replacement), has made going to the bathroom as clean and swift as firing a tennis ball gun! This dramatic difference really helped to highlight that what you think is a normal, healthy experience in the bathroom, may, in actual fact, be nothing of the sort.

As a result, I have included the "SuperGreens" and "Super Berry"formulas in the Survivors Guide cheat sheet towards the end of this book. It really is that good.

If you would like more information, I have written an article on it here:

http://www.CancerUncensored.com/living-fuel

(Men) Sit down to use the toilet

Whilst on the topic, it is worth mentioning that men have a higher risk of bowel cancer than women. Part of this is believed to be the fact that they do not sit down to use the toilet when they urinate.

I have noticed that sitting to urinate has, on numerous occasions, triggered a bowel movement that I had no idea was there. Had I been standing at the urinal, as most men do, that waste material would be still on board, increasing my risk of bowel cancer.

This simple change in habit can help to address the increased risk that men live under for this particular form of cancer. It is unfair to isolate this change in habit as being the only contributory factor, because men do tend to consume more red meat than women, but nevertheless a strategy to address both factors would be optimum.

Increasing your daily fibre intake has been shown to significantly reduce bowel cancer risk for both sexes.

Dry skin brushing

In Western medicine and Western society, we are very guilty of compartmentalising our bodies and not treating them as an interconnected system. Doctors tend to treat symptoms and not causes.

For example, we should view a tumour as a symptom of a larger condition. The tumour itself is a manifestation of our system breaking down. If we target the cause, (such as poor diet), and change the inputs into our system, we give it a fighting chance to correct itself through the natural inbuilt processes that normally keep you cancer-free.

It is the same way with how we view our organs. The narrow view is that each organ has its own unique function. Your brain allows you to think, your heart pumps blood around your body, your kidneys eliminate waste, and so on.

However, given that our body is a complex interconnected system, it isn't accurate to assume that a single function is catered for by a single organ.

A good illustration of this, is the fact that your skin actually eliminates a quarter of the toxins from the body. It is sometimes referred to as the third kidney. Your lungs are sometimes referred to as the second kidney. Each has the capacity to help our bodies eliminate waste and toxins. If one organ is overloaded, the others are able to assist.

The skin is the largest organ in the body, with its primary role being to keep the external environment out. However, its secondary function is the elimination of up to 1 lb of waste acids and toxins per day!

Poor circulation, sluggish movement of your lymphatic system, blocked pores and a range of other issues hamper your skin's ability to support your kidneys. This can often be evidenced by acne, hives, body odour, itchiness, rashes and even eczema or psoriasis.

If toxins are not allowed, or are unable, to escape through your skin, they become trapped in your fat tissues, contributing to cellulite. Alternatively, they are reabsorbed into your bloodstream, which adds to the strain on your liver and kidneys.

This is where dry skin brushing comes in. Many people consider dry skin brushing to be purely a cosmetic process. However, it has been shown to strengthen the immune system, improve our digestion, improve circulation, stimulate the nervous system and improve muscle tone.

With regards to cancer, perhaps the most important aspect of dry skin brushing is improving the flow of the lymph in your lymphatic system.

Your lymphatic system is a vitally important part of your immune system because it enables the movement of white blood cells, called lymphocytes, to carry nutrients to cells and remove waste. Your lymphatic system is independent of your bloodstream, but waste products are removed to the blood, for quicker elimination from the body by the liver and kidneys.

Usually, exercise stimulates the flow of your lymphatic system, when your muscles contract. The lymphatic system has one-way valves that enable the fluid to move when the muscles contract, without then returning to the same point afterwards.

In the absence of exercise or physical stimulation of the skin, lymph may not move quickly enough, resulting in external symptoms such as swollen tissues, e.g. Swollen ankles.

By engaging in dry skin brushing, you are able to get the lymphatic movement your body needs to operate a significant part of your immune system efficiently.

Dry skin brushing also stimulates the hormonal and oil glands. Your skin naturally produces oils that are necessary to stay healthy.

The removal of dead skin cells is also necessary to prevent them from clogging the system. Clogged pores can result in body odour, because sweating is an important part of detoxification. Stimulating the nerve endings in your skin also tones your muscles and tightens the skin.

When you are choosing a brush for dry skin brushing, be sure to buy a natural fibre vegetable bristle brush, because it will not scratch your skin like synthetic brushes can. You also need a brush with a long handle to make it more practical and able to brush your back. If you find the brush to be a little bit course, you can desensitise your skin by conducting this process with a towel until you are used to it.

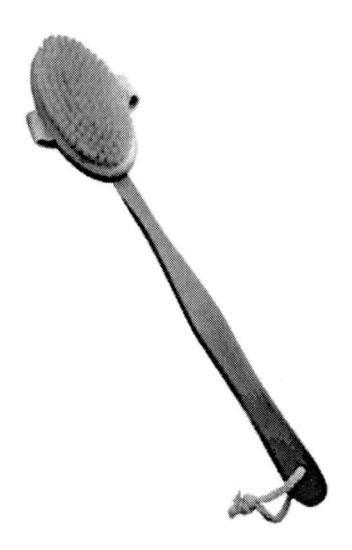

For best results, brush before showering or bathing, but brush yourself at least once per day. The more vigorous you are able to be, the better, but bear in mind that dry skin brushing is different from brushing in the bath, because wet brushing may stretch your skin.

Start with the soles of your feet first, because the nerve endings there can stimulate your whole body. You are always going to brush with long sweeping strokes towards the heart, because this mirrors the motion of your lymphatic system. Avoid brushing areas with broken skin.

Brush your ankles, your calves and thighs, followed by your stomach, buttocks and back.

Brushing your abdomen in clockwise circles, (if you imagine you have a clock face painted on your stomach), may also help to stimulate your digestive system to remove waste products. Brush from your fingers, up your arms, then finally, from your shoulders down your chest towards your heart.

For optimum results, follow your warm bath or shower by a very quick rinse in cool water, because it triggers a change in your blood circulation which may aid in the removal of toxins close to the surface of your skin.

Feel free to spend extra time on hips, thighs and buttocks to help break down cellulite, which may be storing additional toxins that have built up over time. Many people find that doing this process for several months can have dramatic results, both in terms of their health and also in the appearance of their cellulite.

Be sure to clean your brush in water every few weeks, but allow it to dry before you use it again.

Far-Infrared sauna

Infrared sauna is a type of sauna that uses infrared light to generate heat within the skin. A standard sauna heats the air, which in turn, transfers that heat to your body. But infrared sauna heats you up directly.

The infrared light created does not have the potentially damaging rays that sunlight has, purely the component that generates heat. No adverse effects have been reported with infrared sauna, so it is believed to be perfectly safe.

The benefit is that it encourages your body to sweat, (in exactly the same way as when you have a fever), which helps to eliminate toxins from your skin. It also increases your heart rate, and amazingly, can burn as much as 700 calories in an hour whilst you just sit there!

Studies have shown that infrared saunas can have health benefits for those people with high blood pressure, rheumatoid arthritis, congestive heart failure and more, but further studies are required to fully support that data.

Long-term benefits include lower blood pressure, better skin tone, reduced muscle and joint tenderness, faster healing of bruises, cuts and acne, an increased level of weight loss, reduced stress, deeper sleep and more.

Perhaps most importantly, infrared sauna enables those people who have recently undertaken major surgery to get the benefits of mild exercise without actually having to physically exercise, which may put stress on their bodies and hinder their recovery.

With regard to cancer, the additional elimination of toxins may help your body to function correctly, thereby giving you the maximum chance of recovery, or remaining well. The increased circulation also increases the oxygenation of your tissues, which creates an environment that is more hostile to cancer cells. Finally, the artificial fever condition created in the body is more hostile to cancer cells than healthy tissue, because cancer cells do not tolerate heat as well.

Clearly, diet, exercise and eliminating exposure to toxins will have a greater impact, but infrared sauna can play a part in the bigger picture of your health.

Meditation

Meditation involves calming the mind and body in order to relieve anxiety, stress, pain and to focus your body's resources on healing.

The connection between mind and body has been indisputably proven, but the mechanism by which it works is simply not understood. Equally, harnessing the tremendous benefits is a matter of personal practice and perseverance.

Since the 1950s, over 3000 studies on meditation have been conducted, including studies on visualisation, which showed that sports people could achieve greater improvement in their game or sport through visualisation than control groups who simply practised the sport.

Dr Herbert Benson, founder of the Mind-Body Medical Institute, which is affiliated with Harvard University, has documented that meditation induces a wide range of biochemical and physical changes, which he collectively referred to as the "relaxation response". These changes include altered respiration, heart rate, blood pressure, metabolism, response to pain and brain chemistry.

Given that stress actively increases your body's amount of circulating free radicals, and free radicals are linked to an increase in the rate of cancer, it follows that eliminating stress through meditation should directly impact upon your level of cancer risk if engaged in on a regular basis.

A study conducted by Yale, Harvard, and Massachusetts General Hospital has demonstrated that meditation actively increases the volume of grey matter in certain parts of your brain. Using brain scans and participants with intensive Buddhist "insight meditation" training, alongside a control group who did not meditate, the researchers discovered that the parts of the brain responsible for processing sensory input and attention span had increased thickness.

The researchers concluded that it may be possible to use meditation as a measure to slow the deterioration of brain tissue in later life.

With regard to cancer, in 2006, researchers reviewed the findings of nine different studies on mindfulness meditation and cancer. The findings were that practising mindfulness meditation yielded "consistent benefits", including an improvement in stress levels, the ability to cope, psychological functioning, pain management, fatigue, sleep patterns, mood and general well-being.

Another controlled study of mindfulness meditation showed that those who meditated had an improved immune response to the influenza vaccine than those who did not meditate. So if mindfulness meditation can measurably improve immune response, surely it can play a part in cancer prevention and cancer treatment.

In light of this, I feel that meditation is a valuable addition to your toolbox. Of course, it does not replace lifestyle changes, improvement in your diet and medical treatment, but it is a worthy addition.

The only caveat is that meditation may not be suitable for you if you have mental illness. If this applies to you, please consult with your Doctor.

To discover up-to-date resources relating to guided meditation, visit:

http://www.CancerUncensored.com/meditation

Socialising

As you will see from the Psychology section of this book, you should never underestimate the power of the mind to influence your health and wellbeing.

Dr Lisa Berkman, of the Harvard School of Health Sciences, reported the results of a nine-year study of 7000 people aged 35 to 65. She noted that people who lacked social and community ties were almost 3 times more likely to die of medical illness than those with more extensive contacts. This was independent from socio-economic status and health practices, such as smoking, alcohol consumption, obesity and physical activity.

Find excuses to expand your social circle, and to be around positive people. Laughter has also been shown to have a positive impact, along with being married, (and the nurturing support structure it creates).

Environmental Factors to Avoid

This section details a range of known factors that can contribute towards your risk of cancer. If you can avoid these factors, you will decrease your risk, or if you have already been diagnosed, avoiding these factors will ease the burden placed on your body whilst you are fighting the disease.

Smoking (or use of tobacco in any form)

Smoking is undoubtedly the most well-known cause of cancer. However, it wasn't always so. It took years to prove and there was a lot of resistance to it because of the huge amounts of money at stake.

Smoking is responsible for 1 in 4 deaths from cancer in the UK and kills more people than murder, suicide, road accidents, drug overdoses and HIV put together. It is entirely preventable.

Whilst lung cancer is what most people associate with smoking, the cocktail of numerous carcinogenic chemicals in each cigarette can trigger cancers of the mouth, nose and sinuses, larynx (voice box), pharynx (upper throat), the oesophagus, stomach, bowel, liver, pancreas, kidney, bladder, cervix, ovaries, breasts, prostate and blood (leukaemia).

Clearly the best option is to quit smoking and to avoid exposure of passive smoking.

Failing that, if stopping smoking is not an option, then certain dietary changes may help to reduce your risk

As I mentioned in the Hazelnut section of this book, According to the Journal of the National Cancer Institute, a government study of nearly 30,000 men showed that vitamin E supplements (taken at 400 IU per day), cut the prostate Cancer risk for smokers by 71%.

Another study published in the International Journal of Cancer in 2008, highlighted the significant differences in effectiveness of different kinds of vitamin E. There are four different kinds of Tocopherol (vitamin E) - alpha, beta, gamma and delta. The study found that increasing alpha-tocopherol consumption to 7.73mg per day or greater resulted in a 34 to 53% reduction in lung cancer risk. Beta, gamma and delta tocopherols did not have the same dramatic effect. So if you do supplement with vitamin E, make sure it is the alpha-tocopherol you are using.

You can find a list of foods containing apha-tocopherol, and many other nutrients using the nutrition finder at:

http://www.CancerUncensored.com/nutrient-search

or

http://nutritiondata.self.com/tools/nutrient-search

But for the sake of clarity, my advice is to please stop smoking, do not rely on a magic pill or a vitamin in food.

Wearing a bra?

Whilst there has been the bare minimum of publicity about it, it could be argued that bras are as significant to breast cancer as smoking is to lung cancer.

In the book "Dressed to Kill" by medical anthropologists Sydney Ross Singer and Soma Grismaijer, study data was put forward as compelling evidence that bras may have a dramatic impact upon breast cancer rates.

Singer and Grismaijer noticed that in cultures where women were "bra-free", women had similar breast cancer rates to men. The Maori of New Zealand, Aboriginals of Australia, Fijians and Japanese who did not wear bras all had exceptionally low breast cancer levels. Even more compelling was that when these cultures were "Westernised" and women started wearing bras, they ended up with breast cancer rates equivalent to Western women.

Singer and Grismaijer conducted a study on over 4,700 US women across five major US cities. Approximately half of the women involved in the study had previously been diagnosed with breast cancer. The study determined what bra wearing habits these women had, and in particular, their behaviour prior to diagnosis.

The study data indicated that the longer you wear your bra each day, the greater the likelihood of your developing breast cancer.

They reported that:

- 3 out of 4 women who wore their bras 24 hours per day developed breast cancer.
- 1 out of 7 women who wore bras more than 12 hour per day, (but not to bed), developed breast cancer.
- 1 out of 152 women who wore their bras less than 12 hours per day got breast cancer.
- Only 1 out of 168 women who wore bras rarely (or never) were diagnosed with breast cancer.

Unfortunately, the US National Cancer Institute, the American Cancer Society, and the US National Institute of Health all refused to acknowledge this data. This is despite other studies that have offered supporting evidence, such as a study of 3,918 cases of breast cancer and 11,712 controls from seven centres in the United States.

This particular study found that premenopausal women who did not wear bras only had half the level of risk of breast cancer, compared with women who did wear bras.

The opposing argument was that typically, those women who do not wear bras have smaller breasts and are thinner. Therefore, breast size could be used as an indicator of cancer risk, rather than the presence, or absence of a bra.

Whilst we cannot say for certain what the truth of the matter is without further research, I believe this data is an excellent starting point for further study.

If this data is valid, it is vitally important, because many women have absolutely no idea that their bra could be so detrimental to their health.

Singer and Grismaijer believed that the trigger for the increase in cancer risk was the fact that bras restricted the flow of fluids within the lymphatic system, leading to a buildup of fluid within breast tissue. They hypothesised that toxins in the lymphatic system could collect in the breast lymphatic vessels due to the constriction caused by the bra. The concentration of these toxins within the breast tissue could then ultimately lead to cancer.

According to Dr David Williams MD, "wearing a bra at least 14 hours a day tends to increase the hormone prolactin, which decreases circulation in the breast tissue. Decreasing circulation can impede your body's natural removal of carcinogenic fluids that become trapped in the breast's sac-like glands (lymphnodes). These glands make up the largest mass of lymph nodes in the upper part of your body's lymphatic system."

I think this data is compelling enough to certainly avoid wearing a bra if you have been diagnosed with breast cancer. If you haven't, then you should still perhaps limit your use of one. Certainly, further study should be undertaken, but sadly it appears that none of the cancer research organisations are even looking into it, having dismissed it out of hand.

If you were cynical, you might wonder if the multibillion turnover of the brassiere and fashion industry, or multibillion chemotherapy and radiotherapy spend on breast cancer had anything to do with it. You can read more on the biases of the cancer research community in the Cancer Research section of this book.

Excessive sun exposure or excessive suntan lotion exposure?

As I mentioned in the Anticancer Activities section of this book, moderate sun exposure has substantial advantages. However, conventional "wisdom" dictates that skin cancer is a very real risk if you are not adequately protected or perhaps if you spend too much time in the sun.

According to mainstream medicine, the key is to make sure that you do not actually burn. Try not to spend any more than half an hour in the sun at any one time, use suntan lotion with a high SPF factor, (minimum 15), and take a hat with you if you are likely to be out in the sun for longer than half an hour. This is particularly important for people with a fair or pale complexion.

Most importantly, become very familiar with your skin so that you can spot any changes over time. In the Early Detection section of this book, I give detailed information on how to perform regular self examinations.

Symptoms to look out for are:

- A small lump on your skin that can be smooth or waxy in appearance. It may bleed sometimes or develop a crust.
- A flat red spot which can become scaly or crusty.
- A firm, red lump.
- A hard, horny lump that is tender to the touch.

Ironically, some health experts now warn that suntan lotions contain toxic chemicals that can do more harm than good, whilst also reducing the oxygen absorption of your skin, so it is very difficult to know whether it is the lotion or the sun that is more dangerous.

A notable study conducted in Australia showed that lifeguards, who are in the sun all day, get less skin cancers than office workers, who only get intermittent exposure. So perhaps the link isn't so much due to sun exposure, but also that exercise levels and diet impact your susceptibility to it? Or perhaps people who work indoors tend to burn themselves when they do get time in the sun?

The Environmental Working Group, (EWG), have found that only around 8% of suntan lotions are both safe and effective for the intended use, whereas the other 92 percent contain at least one (if not many more) of the ingredients designated as detrimental for human use!

In the BMJ, (British Medical Journal), Dr Sam Shuster argues that 75% of melanomas occur on relatively unexposed areas of the body, that incidence and mortality FALL with greater exposure and that the incidence is unaffected or even INCREASED with the use of sunscreens.

Radon gas

Radon is a form of radioactive gas that can sometimes gather in people's homes. It is formed by the elemental decay of uranium, radium, and thorium in soil and rock. Depending on the foundations of your property and upon what material it rests, radon can seep up through the ground and diffuse into the air.

If your home does not have adequate ventilation, and is in an area prone to radon, you may get a buildup.

Unfortunately, radon is invisible, and odourless, so you can only detect it using a simple home test kit.

Whilst radon does not often make the headlines, it is the second most common cause of lung cancer, killing between 15,000 and 22,000 people every year in the US.

Basements and ground floors of well insulated and tightly sealed homes may be susceptible to the highest level of buildup, so take the time to ventilate your home regularly. Not only will this limit your exposure to radon, but it will also improve the oxygen levels.

In the US, the Environmental Protection Agency recommends that homes should have a radon level below 4 picocuries per litre (4 pCi/L) of air. An estimated 1 in 15 homes has radon levels exceeding this level.

Read more about simple home test kits for radon at:

http://www.CancerUncensored.com/radon-test-kits

Radiation and magnetic fields

Mobile Telephones

The World Health Organisation has placed mobile phones (cellphones) into the category of "possibly carcinogenic".

An advisory panel, the International Agency for Research on Cancer, reviewed numerous existing studies focused on the health effects of radio frequency magnetic fields, which are emitted by mobile phones. They concluded that heavy cellphone usage increased the risk of a rare type of brain cancer called glioma.

In 2010, the largest and longest study of its kind, spanning 13 countries, called Interphone, determined that participants with the highest level of mobile phone use had a 40% greater risk of glioma. In fairness, gliomas are quite rare, so they do not increase your overall cancer risk greatly. However, a risk is a risk, so this has been included for you to be able to make your own informed choices about mobile phone use.

Using a Bluetooth headset, hands-free kit or speakerphone, so that you are further away from the actual source of radiation would certainly be advisable whilst you are speaking on the phone.

The classification given to mobile phones of "possibly carcinogenic", Category 2B, contains over 240 other items, including the pesticide DDT, vehicle exhaust fumes, various industrial chemicals, lead, pickled vegetables and coffee.

Power Lines

Power lines create an electromagnetic field (EMF). Electrical devices within the home can create a small electromagnetic field, but industrial power lines create a field of much greater magnitude. Of course, the link between power lines and cancer is hotly disputed, possibly due to the potential magnitude of liability.

As the voltage increases, so does the strength of the electromagnetic field, so high-voltage cables have a greater potential to penetrate the body.

A number of studies have focused upon magnetic field exposure and the risk of cancer in children. Given that the two most common forms of cancer amongst children are brain tumours and leukaemia, the majority of the research has concentrated on these.

In 1979, one notable study highlighted a possible association between living near electric power lines and the incidence of childhood leukaemia. More recent studies have had mixed findings. Some have found an association whilst others have not.

When researchers combined nine well conducted studies, from several different countries, (which included a study from the National Cancer Institute), a twofold increase in the risk of childhood leukaemia was linked to exposure to magnetic fields greater than 0.4 µT (0.4 microtesla).

When 15 other studies were combined, similar results were found at magnetic field levels above 0.3 µT (0.3 microtesla)

On that basis, if you live under, or very near to, substantial electrical power lines, it is worth investigating whether you are being influenced by a magnetic field. Whilst the studies only focused on brain cancer and leukemia, I would not rule out other forms of cancer, or other health influences.

After all, a study published in the Journal of the National Institute of Environmental Health Sciences, showed that although extremely low frequency electromagnetic fields (ELF-EMF) did not directly cause DNA damage or mutations in their experiments, they did influence the way that genes were expressed in leukaemia cells. Via a magnetic field, they were able to trigger the proliferation of leukaemia cells.

The researchers stated that they were not able to create cancer, however, they were able to switch genes "on and off at inappropriate times, causing these initiated cells to proliferate when normally they would just sit there quietly doing nothing."

In addition, two studies published in the American Journal of Epidemiology indicated increased risk of breast cancer associated with magnetic fields. One Norwegian study, published in 2004, found an elevation of risk due to exposure to magnetic fields in the home. The second study, published in 2003, detailed an increased risk in breast cancer for African-American women using electric bedding. (If you use an electric blanket, just use it to heat your bed up, then switch it off before you get in).

To test your home, you can buy an electromagnetic field meter or Tesla meter from eBay for between £50 to £100 or US $80 to $150. Just make sure it can read in microtesla (μT).

CT scans, x-rays and mammograms

"... About 75% of the current annual incidence of breast cancer in the US is being caused by earlier ionising radiation, primarily from medical sources." - John W. Gofman, M.D.

The truth is, we do not know the cause of breast cancer for certain. Indeed, there are likely several factors at play, but medical radiation is certainly a known and contributory risk factor.

A 1993 Swedish study involving over 42,000 women highlighted that those women under the age of 55 who received premenopausal mammography experienced a 29% greater risk of dying from breast cancer.

A study published in 2012 in the New England Journal of Medicine has highlighted the fact that mammograms can be responsible for a substantial level of overdiagnosis. The study claims that 1.3 million women have been incorrectly diagnosed, or overdiagnosed, with breast cancer in the last 30 years. This represents 31% of breast cancer diagnosis. This means that almost a third of the women treated would not actually have become sick in the first place, had they been left alone.

Due to the extensive use of radiation in modern medical imaging techniques, our average lifetime exposure to radiation has almost doubled since 1980. In fact, studies show that medical radiation accounts for just over half of our total lifetime radiation exposure.

The FDA are taking steps to limit patients' exposure to medical radiation by the stricter regulation of CT scans, but have not addressed the dangers of mammography.

CT scans have become an invaluable part of modern medicine, helping doctors to diagnose more accurately. CT scans can be used to gain a cross-section image of any part of your body, allowing doctors to evaluate trauma, abdominal pain, seizures and a range of other ailments.

However, as useful as they are, a single chest CT scan can expose you to as much radiation as nearly 400 chest x-rays! (A total of 0.4 rads). As a result, almost all medical societies recommend minimising your exposure to medical radiation.

This message doesn't always reach patients, so you need to be sure to question your Doctor if they recommend a CT scan. Is it absolutely necessary?

The chairman of the Cancer Prevention Coalition, Samuel S Epstein MD, commended the FDA for warning the public about the radiation from CT scans, but said that "the FDA remains strangely unaware that radiation from routine premenopausal mammography poses significant and cumulative risk of breast cancer."

Given that it is routine practice to take two films of each breast during mammography, and that the radiation is directed at a very small section of tissue, instead of being spread across a large area, this results in an exposure of approximately 0.4 rads - the same as a CT scan in each breast.

Dr Epstein further explained "Thus, premenopausal women undergoing annual screening over a ten-year period are exposed to a total of at least 4 rads for each breast, at least 8 times greater radiation than FDA's "cancer risk" level."

"Such high radiation exposure approximates to that of Japanese women living approximately 1 mile away from the site of the

Hiroshima atom bomb explosion."

In 1972, the National Academy of Sciences warned that the total risk of breast cancer increases by 1% for every 1 rad of exposure. By their estimates, this totals a 10% greater risk from 10 years annual premenopausal mammography, but by Dr Epstein's estimates this could be as much as 40%.

As a result, in Dr. Epstein's book, "The Politics of Cancer", he states, "Whatever you may be told, refuse routine mammograms, especially if you are pre-menopausal. The x-rays may increase your chances of getting cancer."

Even if you do not agree with Dr Epstein's recommendations, there are things you can do right now to reduce your radiation exposure. For example, instead of mammography, opt for thermography.

Thermography, (thermal imaging), is a completely harmless alternative to mammography and is available to many women for around £180 or $280.

Whilst in some countries it hasn't yet gained mainstream approval, it works by accurately detecting hot spots in breast tissue, which are consistent with the presence of tumours.

I would recommend it as a solid alternative to the ionising radiation from mammography. If your doctor cannot refer you to a local centre who can conduct thermography, then you should search the Internet for your nearest location.

Early detection is still vitally important, but it should not be compromised by the damaging effects of radiation.

Known conditions that contribute to cancer risk

There are a range of health conditions and diseases which can increase your risk of cancer. If you address these, you should no longer be at an elevated level of risk.

For example, the American Cancer Association estimate that 14 to 20% of all cancer deaths are related to obesity.

If you lose the weight, you reduce your level of cancer risk. If weight is an issue for you, consider a wheat-free diet, avoiding high fructose corn syrup and including whey protein and almonds, which both chemically induce a feeling of satiety after eating.

Other conditions that increase your risk include: (This list is not exhaustive).

- Human papillomavirus (HPV)
- Chlamydia
- Stomach ulcers
- Helicobacter pylori
- Bulemia
- Sleep apnoea
- Hormone replacement therapy
- High body mass index (BMI)
- Ovarian cysts
- Endometriosis
- Hepatitis B or C
- Cirrhosis of the liver
- Diabetes
- Pancreatitis
- HIV

Diesel/petrol and exhaust fumes

It is estimated that around 5% of cancer is related to pollution. Vehicle exhaust fumes have been on the World Health

Organisation's list of possible carcinogens for a while, but as of 2012 they were upgraded to "carcinogenic to humans", so you should avoid them where possible.

The World Health Organisation panel of experts concluded that exhaust fumes were definitely a cause of lung cancer and may also cause bladder tumours. These findings were based on research following high-risk workers such as truck drivers, railway workers and miners.

If you work in a high risk industry (with exposure to exhaust fumes), it is estimated that you have a 40% increased risk of developing lung cancer.

Equally, when fuelling your vehicle, it is worth wearing the disposable gloves that are provided on the garage forecourt.

If you don't believe that you are coming into contact with diesel or petrol when you fill your vehicle, sniff your hand after you next fill your tank!

Carcinogens

"We are all so contaminated that if we were cannibals, our meat would be banned from human consumption." - Paula Baillie-Hamilton, M.D.

Every year a freely available "Report on Carcinogens" is published by the US National Toxicology Program, which lists all known carcinogens. This can be freely downloaded from the Internet.

The 12th edition, published in 2011, states "The probability that a resident of the United States will develop cancer at some point in his or her lifetime is 1 in 2 for men and 1 in 3 for women (ACS 2010). Nearly everyone's life has been directly or indirectly affected by cancer. Most scientists involved in cancer research believe that the environment in which we live and work may be a major contributor to the development of cancer (Lichtenstein et al. 2000). In this context, the "environment" is anything that people interact with, including exposures resulting from lifestyle choices, such as what we eat, drink, or smoke; natural and medical radiation, including exposure to sunlight; workplace exposures; drugs; socioeconomic factors that affect exposures and susceptibility; and substances in air, water, and soil (OTA 1981, IOM 2001). Other factors that play a major role in cancer development are infectious diseases, aging, and individual susceptibility, such as genetic predisposition (Montesano and Hall 2001). We rarely know what environmental factors and conditions are responsible for the onset and development of cancer; however, we have some understanding of how some types of cancer develop, especially cancer related to certain occupational exposures or the use of specific drugs. Many experts firmly believe that much of the cancer associated with the environment may be avoided (Tomatis et al. 1997)."

Many of the most prominent carcinogenic substances are listed in this book, but of course it is not exhaustive. The report on carcinogens is where you can get more information on known cancer risk factors.

Aluminium-based antiperspirants and deodorants (US spelling - Aluminum)

Aluminium salts (aluminum salts) are the active antiperspirant ingredient used in many underarm deodorants.

Mainstream cancer research organisations claim that there is no link between these antiperspirants and breast cancer. However, recent studies indicate otherwise.

Aluminium-based antiperspirants work by blocking the pores of your underarms, preventing the release of sweat. However, this also blocks the release of toxins from your lymphatic system.

These toxins do not disappear, they are simply left as deposits in the lymph nodes below the arms. Such a concentration of toxins can lead to cell mutation. Is it a coincidence that most breast tumours occur in the upper outside quadrant of the breast area, which is where lymph nodes are located?

A study published in the Journal of Applied Toxicology showed that not only is the aluminium preventing your excretion of toxins, it is also being absorbed by your body and deposited in the breast tissue. The study even showed that aluminium can be detected in nipple aspirate fluid, which is found in the breast duct tree.

The researchers discovered that the average level of aluminium in nipple aspirate fluid was significantly higher in those women who had been affected by breast cancer, compared with healthy women. Aluminium is not normally present in the body, so testing for aluminium in nipple aspirate fluid may be a useful indicator of higher breast cancer risk.

A 2007 study, published in the Journal of Inorganic Biochemistry, which analysed breast tissue samples from cancer patients who had undergone mastectomies, showed that the women who used antiperspirants had deposits of aluminium in their outer breast tissue.

Animal studies have shown that aluminium can cause cancer, and we know that aluminium salts can mimic the hormone oestrogen, which can increase breast cancer risk, particularly in postmenopausal women.

Many commercial brands of antiperspirant contain either aluminium zirconium, or aluminium chlorohydrate, which is very water-soluble and is readily absorbed by the body. Once in the body, the molecule ionises, forming an aluminium free radical. This free radical can pass across cell membranes and can be selectively absorbed by the liver, bone marrow, cartilage, kidneys and brain, making it not only a concern for breast cancer, but also Alzheimer's disease.

Whilst the data has yet to be embraced by mainstream cancer research organisations, you have the power to opt for a deodorant which does not contain aluminium salts.

When reading the label, avoid products containing aluminum chlorohydrate, aluminum chloride, aluminum hydroxybromide or aluminum zirconium.

I have recently purchased a product called "terra NATURALS" which does not contain any aluminium, propylene glycol, steareth 100, steareth 20, polysorbate 20, triclosan, ethylhexylglycerine or parabens. Instead, it uses a sugar-based odour control, with immune supplements, prebiotics and lymph cleansing herbs. Learn more at:

http://www.CancerUncensored.com/recommended-products

Allergens / food intolerances

This section is geared towards people who may not even know they are intolerant or allergic to certain foods or environmental factors. It is estimated that over 54% of Americans have allergies.

But the information in this section does not necessarily apply to the 15% of the population who may have dangerous allergies or anaphylaxis.

Clearly, if you are so allergic to something that it causes your throat to swell, causes you to feel faint, dizzy, nauseous or have a rapid pulse, along with wheezing, hives and itching, then you have more pressing concerns than its long-term effects on your cancer risk.

In those susceptible, such a drastic reaction can be related to foods, including peanuts, shellfish, eggs, milk, wheat, tree nuts, soy and fish. Alternatively, insect stings, different drugs or latex can be a trigger.

If you are having any such reaction, please consult a doctor immediately.

With that said, there is conflicting information available on the impact that food intolerances or allergies have on your risk of cancer.

It appears to be related largely to the type and duration of the allergic response. In short, it appears that extended exposure to allergens has a negative impact, whilst brief and limited exposure appears to have a potentially positive impact.

This is perhaps due to the difference between the short-term activation of your immune system, versus the longer-term and sustained **exhaustion** of your immune system.

An article published in the Journal of the American Medical Association, which analysed data collected from 1969 to 2008, followed 30,000 sufferers of coeliac disease. Coeliac disease is a chronic and severe form of gluten intolerance that affects approximately 1 in 100 people in the US. Less severe symptoms are visible in as many as a third of the US population, hence my recommendation to avoid wheat.

The research showed that wheat and gluten intolerance isn't just restricted to causing gastric disturbances, it can also have an impact upon your risk of heart disease, cancer and premature death.

The study divided participants into three groups: those with gluten sensitivity, those with intestinal inflammation but not full-blown coeliac disease, and those diagnosed with coeliac disease.

The study discovered that having a long-term persistent allergic reaction significantly increased the likelihood of death. Those with gluten sensitivity had a 35% higher risk of death, those with full-blown coeliac disease had a 39% increased risk, and for those individuals with intestinal inflammation, there was a 72% increased risk of death.

Many people have a gluten intolerance, but they are not aware that this is the cause of their symptoms. Irritable bowel disease is more obvious, but other symptoms may include osteoporosis, rheumatoid arthritis, lupus, anaemia, MS, autoimmune disease and cancer.

There is a particularly high correlation with lymphoma, which is a cancer of the immune system. There is also a correlation between neurological problems and gluten intolerance, including autism, epilepsy, schizophrenia, depression, anxiety, migraines and dementia.

If you don't think this affects you, then look again. A study of blood tests, which compared 10,000 blood tests from 50 years ago to 10,000 tests conducted on people today, showed a 400% increase in full-blown coeliac disease. With many more samples also showing elevated TTG antibodies, which appear when your body is having a reaction to gluten.

The most common symptoms include undiagnosed skin rashes and digestive disturbances, but it is not always obvious.

Gluten is contained in a number of grains, not just wheat, so if you are gluten intolerant, you should also avoid barley, rye, oats and more. Gluten is even found in beer, some cosmetics, some vitamin tablets, some salad dressings, some soups, etc.

Avoiding gluten will take more information and guidance than is provided in this book, so please seek medical advice if this affects you. Certainly, you can request a gluten intolerance test from your Doctor.

With regard to other allergies, such as contact allergies, a study of over 17,000 adults by the National Allergy Research Centre in Copenhagen showed that those who had contact allergies were statistically less likely to develop cancer in later life than those who did not have allergies.

The researchers successfully used data from Denmark's National Cancer Registry, which recorded every single case of diagnosed cancer since 1943.

Approximately one third of the participants tested positive to contact allergies, when researchers exposed a small patch of their skin to various allergens.

The lead researcher, Kaare Engkilde, explained that "People with allergies seem to have less cancer or have fewer different cancer types than patients who don't have allergies."

"The reason for this is uncertain but it might have to do with the immune surveillance theory, which speculates that patients with allergies may have a more ready and observant immune system that could lead to earlier detection of cancerous cells."

Given that allergic reactions are basically a heightened immune response to foreign compounds, such as dust, pet fur, nickel or other agents, those individuals with allergies may have an immune system that is already on high alert for any foreign materials or indeed tumours.

However, whilst having contact allergies correlated with reducing cancer risk overall, (with particular emphasis on skin and breast cancers), not every type of cancer was negatively affected. There was an increase in the likelihood of bladder cancer.

Perhaps the most comprehensive review of the relationship between allergies and cancer has been conducted by Cornell University, which evaluated the data from well over 600 previous studies.

The research team discovered that not only did it vary from one allergy to another, but the relationship varied depending on the type of allergic reaction. Most importantly, they questioned the approach of inhibiting the symptoms of allergy, which is very common in modern medicine.

They discovered that the allergic reaction helped the body to eliminate toxins and remove the allergen.

For example, sneezing, runny nose and watering eyes all help to cleanse your system, removing the allergen that triggered the reaction. Suppressing the symptoms does not deal with the problem, it simply masks it.

They found that organs which had direct contact with the environmental particles that caused the allergy, actually had the least amount of cancer in those people with allergies. These included the mouth, throat, colon, rectum, cervix, pancreas and glial brain cells.

Tissues that were more isolated from allergens, such as prostate, breast or meningeal brain cells did not show a reduction in incidence.

There are always exceptions to the rule, however.

Unfortunately, asthma sufferers did suffer from higher rates of lung cancer, because the "asthma obstructs clearance of pulmonary mucous, blocking any potential benefit of allergic expulsion". But other lung-related allergies did show protective effects.

The research team were very clear that if allergic response is the body's natural defence against disease and foreign materials, then why would switching off this mechanism via artificial intervention be a good idea?

Yes, we get the short-term relief from the symptoms, but a runny nose, cough or skin breakout is just your body's way of eliminating toxins and unwanted materials.

So what does this mean to you?

Well, I believe that knowledge is power, so having yourself tested for food intolerances and allergies gives you a good starting point.

After all, for many people, (but not those with dangerous allergies), the occasional exposure to an allergen appears to be relatively harmless or even beneficial, but long-term persistent exposure is clearly detrimental to your health.

When you have your allergy test results, you can avoid inadvertently exposing yourself to something you are intolerant to on a daily basis, such as gluten, as this can negatively impact upon your cancer risk and health.

For more information on allergy testing, visit:

http://www.CancerUncensored.com/allergy-testing

Illegal Drugs

To be fair, both legal and illegal drugs have been shown to be potentially carcinogenic, so I am not specifically singling out illegal drugs. Just look at tobacco as an example.

However, recent studies have shown a significant increase in testicular cancer amongst cannabis / marijuana users.

Testicular cancer is the most common form of cancer found in young men aged 15 to 45, and regular recreational use of cannabis / marijuana doubles your risk according to research conducted by the Keck School of Medicine at the University of Southern Carolina.

In a report released in June 2012, by the British Lung Foundation, which referenced the 2008 study, "Cannabis use and risk of lung cancer: a case-control study" (Aldington et al), published in the European Respiratory Journal, they claimed that a single deeply inhaled joint caused as much lung tissue damage as a whole packet of 20 cigarettes.

Of course, this is hotly disputed by advocates of cannabis use. Lung cancer risk factors aside, research conducted over a 30 year period by King's College London and Duke University in the US, found that cannabis use during adolescence reduces a person's IQ by an average of eight points, and impacts upon their attention span and memory.

Although the link between cannabis use and mental health is not a new one. Heavy cannabis use has been associated with paranoia, schizophrenia, depression, insomnia and a range of other personality and anxiety disorders.

Another drug that could potentially lead to cancer is the use of cocaine cut with impurities. Cocaine is being increasingly frequently cut with Phenacetin, a drug that was banned in many countries in the 1980s due to the fact that it was proven to cause serious kidney damage or cancer.

In the UK, the purity of cocaine has been dropping over the last few years. Current street cocaine purity levels range between 9 and 20% so you never know what you are putting into your body. Even if the cocaine is pure, whilst it does not cause cancer, you still run the risk of a swollen and enlarged heart muscle, nose bleeds and long-term addiction.

As with many other facets of life, I fully appreciate that people have a right to make their own choices. The use of illegal drugs is no exception, but it does carry consequences.

Just in the same way that I would advocate a reduction in coffee consumption, or the elimination of tobacco smoke, I would advocate that you avoid both alcohol consumption and illegal drug use if you are looking toward the best interests of your health.

Dental toxicity

Dental toxicity refers to the impact of mercury-based amalgam fillings, nickel crowns and root canals.

Mercury is more toxic than arsenic, so why does the dental profession think it a good idea to put this into our children's mouths?

Around 10 years ago, I had the mercury fillings in my teeth removed and replaced with white fillings. My dentist had us both use breathing apparatus during the removal for our safety.

The list of symptoms from mercury poisoning is so extensive, that I was unable to list them all here. Central nervous system symptoms ranged from emotional instability through to depression and suicidal tendencies. But the full range of symptoms extended through head, neck and oral cavity disorders, gastrointestinal effects, cardiovascular effects, immunological issues all the way through to kidney, thyroid and adrenal diseases.

Is it any wonder, with all the mercury used in dental practice, that dentists have the highest divorce and suicide rates among professionals? Female dental personnel have an increased incidence of premature labour, increased spontaneous abortion rate and a raised level of perinatal mortality.

It is estimated that 40 tons of mercury is used every year in the US to prepare amalgam fillings. Unfortunately, it is also estimated that each amalgam filling can release as much as 10 micrograms of mercury into the body every day.

"I don't feel comfortable using a substance designated by the Environmental Protection Agency to be a waste disposal hazard. I can't throw it in the trash, bury it in the ground, or put it in a landfill, but they say it is OK to put it in people's mouths. That doesn't make sense." - Richard. Fischer, D.D.S.

"The association of mercury to chronic diseases is well documented in the didactic scientific literature. The search for the association between mercury and cardiovascular disease reveals 358 scientific papers exemplifying the relationship; between mercury and cancer we find 643 scientific papers. The association of mercury with neurodegenerative diseases is the most significant, with the references numbering 1,445." - Dr. Rashid Buttar

The plethora of toxic consequences from mercury must no doubt impact upon your body's ability to fight off cancer. I would suggest that if you have any mercury fillings, you have them removed and replaced with white, non-mercury fillings as I did. I didn't have any obvious symptoms, but understanding the nature of mercury as an adult, I no longer wanted to have them in my mouth.

"Mercury from amalgam fillings has been shown to be neurotoxic, embryotoxic, mutagenic, teratogenic, immunotoxic and clastogenic. It is capable of causing immune dysfunction and auto-immune diseases." "It is estimated that an amalgam filling will release up to half of its mercury content over a ten year period (50% corrosion rate)." - Dr. Robert Gammal

With regard to the dangers of nickel, Thomas Levy, M.D explains "Nickel is rapidly gaining a reputation for its toxicity, too. Most partial dentures are made of nickel. Approximately 80% of crowns use nickel, even "porcelain" crowns. Braces usually are nickel. Stainless steel is usually nickel alloy. Nickel compounds have been unequivocally implicated as human respiratory carcinogens in epidemiological studies of nickel refinery workers, and there appears to be a relationship between nickel crowns and breast cancer in women."

According to Dr. David Eggleston, "Nickel is used routinely by national cancer centers to induce cancer in laboratory animals to study cancer. The nickel alloys they are using are very similar to those we are using in patients' mouths. Dentists are causing a major health problem."

Root Canals are another potential danger to your health.

According to Dr Hal Huggins, D.D.S. in a lecture to the Cancer Control Society 1993. Tape 93F014, "Research has demonstrated that 100% of all root canals result in residual infection due to the imperfect seal that allows bacteria to penetrate. The toxins given off by these bacteria are more toxic than mercury. These toxins can cause systemic diseases of the heart, kidney, uterus, and nervous and endocrine systems."

"The problem with a root canal is that it is dead. Let's equate that. Let's say you have got a ruptured appendix, so you go to the phone book, and who do you look up? Let's see, we have a surgeon and a taxidermist, who do you call? You're going to get it bronzed? That is all we do to a dead tooth. We put a gold crown on it. It looks like it has been bronzed. It doesn't really matter what you embalm the dead tooth with, it is still dead, and within that dead tooth we have bacteria, and these bacteria are in the absence of oxygen. In the absence of oxygen most things die, except bacteria. They undergo something called a pleomorphic change. Like a mutation. They learn to live in the absence of oxygen… Now they produce thioethers, some of the strongest poisons on the planet that are not radioactive. These get out into the body."

"You may notice in the medical literature of 1900 they mentioned a few heart attacks, so it wasn't a big deal in 1900, but by 1910, it was 2% of the US population, which is a lot of folks having heart attacks. By 1920, 10% of the population had had heart attacks, and we are up to about 25% about 10 years ago, and everywhere you go you see joggers running around. Menus in the restaurant have this little heart over it because we are on low cholesterol diets …….so what has it done. It has moved the 25% to around 43%."

"We are going in the wrong direction and root canals are going up. In 1990 we did 17 million of them. This last year we did 23 million, and the ADA hopes by the year 2000 we reach 30 million a year."

"Weston Price knew this back in 1920… He would take a person who had had a heart attack, take out the tooth with the root canal, take a little segment of it, put it under the skin of a rabbit. We have done this with guinea pigs, and in about 10 days that rabbit would die of a heart attack. And you could take it out and put it under the skin of another rabbit, and in 10 days he would die of a heart attack…"

"He would do this to 30 rabbits and every one of them in 97% of the cases would die of heart disease. What if they didn't have heart disease? If they had something else, the rabbit picks up the something else, but all of them that we have tested in this way have ended up with an auto immune disease in the kidney."

"Look at the work of Dr Joseph Issels in Germany, who for 40 years treated terminal cancer cases. He started on them when they had already had their chemo, surgery, radiation, then they came to him. That is having 3 strikes against you and a fast ball down the tube there before you get up to the plate. He turned around 24% of 16,000 patients over a period of 40 years. What is the first thing he did? Have a dentist take out the root canal teeth."

Could dental toxicity be one of many triggers for cancer, and the tumour just be the symptom? If so, removing the mercury, nickel and dead teeth from your mouth could be a solid step toward prevention or even recovery.

Heavy metals

"There is no safe level of mercury, and no one has actually shown that there is a safe level," - Dr. Lars Friberg, Chief Adviser to the WHO on mercury safety.

Lead and aluminium are other common heavy metals that have been repeatedly shown in studies to dramatically increase the toxic effect of mercury.

Medical researchers are still trying to understand the numerous processes by which various heavy metals, (lead, mercury, cadmium, arsenic, chromium, aluminum and more), contribute to carcinogenesis.

For the purposes of cancer prevention however, all we need to know is how to avoid them and how to help remove them from our bodies, as they have a tendency to accumulate.

A good place to start is to filter your drinking water. Please see the Water section in the A-Z of super foods for more information, or visit:

http://www.CancerUncensored.com/water-filters

Eating organic food is also a good strategy, because many heavy metals are used in agriculture and food storage.

Having fat in your diet also helps you to excrete heavy metals. This is another one of the reasons why low-fat diets are not always in your best interests.

Glutathione as a supplement, or eggs, avocado or asparagus can help your body to eliminate heavy metals by acting as antioxidants which minimise the free radicals caused by them.

Whilst fish and seafood are generally a healthy choice, you may inadvertently be consuming heavy metals when you consume them because the seas and rivers are so contaminated. Try to find fish or seafood that has been certified free of mercury and other heavy metals. Ocean caught fish tend to be less contaminated than farmed fish.

Unfortunately, whilst I cannot advocate avoiding vaccines, many vaccines do contain levels of mercury within the preservatives used. Even coloured tattoos are made with ink that is preserved with mercury.

In the US, many homes built prior to 1978, and over 90% of homes built before 1940, contain lead paint. If this applies to you, be sure to either wallpaper over it, or cover it with a thick coating of non-toxic paint.

According to the Campaign for Safe Cosmetics, more than half of the top 33 branded lipsticks contain lead, which is a potent neurotoxin. It has been estimated that the average woman can ingest as much as four pounds of lipstick over the course of her lifetime.

"The latest studies show there is no safe level of lead exposure. Lead builds up in the body over time and lead-containing lipstick applied several times a day, every day, can add up to significant exposure levels." - Mark Mitchell, MD, MPH, director of the Connecticut Coalition for Environmental Justice.

Try to find cosmetics which do not contain any lead or other traces of heavy metals.

Cigarette smoke contains cadmium, so this is another reason to avoid smoking or passive exposure. Cadmium slows down the speed of antibody production in the immune system.

Adding fiber-rich foods to your diet, or foods high in sulphur, such as legumes, onions, eggs and garlic helps the body to rid itself of arsenic, which is a human carcinogen. Arsenic may enter your diet via contaminated drinking water, and some rice, vegetable and cereal products grown on farmland that may have been exposed to it, (due to the use of lead-arsenate insecticides before their ban in the 1980s).

Other than eating healthily, and avoiding sources of heavy metals, your remaining options are to use products such as HMD™, (Heavy Metal Detox - a liquid supplement which is clinically proven to remove / chelate heavy metals from your system), and detox foot pads, which can draw out toxins and heavy metals through your skin overnight.

HMD™ is a 100% natural, effective and safe liquid supplement that costs just over $32 for a month's supply, and has been clinically proven to successfully eliminate lead, antimony, arsenic, cadmium, mercury, nickel, uranium and other toxic metals without eliminating essential minerals. Equally, it does not have any side effects.

It does this by a process called chelation, which is where harmful metals are bound up with peptides, which allows them to be more easily excreted from the body.

In clinical research using a gold-standard double-blind, placebo controlled trial with 350 people, (who worked at a foundry), it was shown that after only a 12-hour provocation with HMD™ there were many heavy metals eliminated in the post-supplement urine and faeces samples, compared with baseline readings. (The following figures are expressed as a % mean increase):

Antimony - 45%
Arsenic - 7,409%
Bismuth - 564%
Cadmium - 67%
Lead - 483%
Mercury - 448%
Nickel - 80%
Uranium - 707%

Incredible results from a product that uses Cilantro Leaf, Homeopathic Chlorella Homaccord and Chlorella Growth Factor (CGF) without any harmful chemicals.

For maximum results, use continuously for 3 months, then maintain the results by using the product for just 1 month each year. HMD™ is safe for all age groups and can be used continuously, but this is not necessary.

Detox foot pads are based upon Japanese medicine. They are a very simple product to use, because you simply apply them to the soles of your feet and then go to bed. In the morning, you find a dark residue on the pad, which has been removed from your system overnight. Over time, the pad gets less and less residue as you clear your system of toxins and heavy metals.

After your initial heavy metal detox, using these pads once per week is more than enough to prevent further accumulation of heavy metals.

For more information on both of these products, visit:

http://www.CancerUncensored.com/recommended-products

"Chelation has not only improved heart disease, stroke, high blood pressure, arthritis, Parkinson's and Alzheimer's disease, but also, studies indicate a 50% reduction in the occurrence of cancer in individuals who have received EDTA! Chelation has been reported to improve asthma, emphysema, brain function, muscular coordination, Multiple Sclerosis and impotence". - From the book Deadly Deception by Dr Willner.

Parasites

"Other prominent physicians agree with me; that in human history, the parasite challenge is likely the most unrecognized of all endemic problems. Because they cannot be seen and rarely present immediate symptoms, they remain invisible as a cause or contributing factor to what can be a serious disorder." - Dr. Ross Andersen, N.D.

Whilst there technically over 3000 different species of parasites, they come in two main categories: microscopic parasites such as single-celled Protozoa and large parasites such as worms.

Microscopic parasites can burrow into your tissues, muscles, bones, joints and organs and feed off your raw materials. Some of them may consume the calcium linings of your bones, or even the coating of your nerves, which can disrupt signals, causing neurological issues. Many parasites also release toxins into your system, which give you a persistent allergy response.

Numerous kinds of worm can inhabit our digestive tract, including pinworms, roundworms, hookworms, tapeworms, threadworms, whipworms and flukes. But it does not stop there, many of these are able to inhabit other tissues in the body such as our liver, lungs, heart, brain, blood, eyes and skin. From thread worms, which measure less than 1 cm in length, up to tapeworms in excess of 30 feet in length.

Despite taking efforts to treat our pets and livestock for worms, we have completely lost sight of the fact that we may well be infested ourselves.

"In terms of numbers there are more parasitic infections acquired in this country than in Africa." - Dr. Frank Nova, Chief of the Laboratory for Parasitic Diseases of the National Institute of Health.

If you have pets, your veterinarian will remind you to worm them regularly, but they do not mention that when your pets groom themselves, any microscopic worm eggs from their faecal matter get licked all over their coat. Then, every time you stroke them, kiss them or share the same furniture with them you risk taking these tiny eggs on board. Many worm species will lay more than 150,000 eggs per day.

If you do not have pets, you will no doubt handle vegetables, eat meat and fish. It is estimated that a square inch cube of sushi can contain as many as 10,000 worm eggs.

Animals, particularly carnivores, have much stronger stomach acid and a shorter digestive tract than we do, so they normally don't have such a problem with worms. However, our bodies can become a mild safe-haven and breeding ground for these parasites.

Incredibly, worms can even influence our mood and appetites to better serve their own ends. If you persistently crave carbohydrates and sugars, it could be an indication that you have worms. It isn't always about the obvious signs, such as an itchy behind.

If you have worms in your intestinal tract, one of the things your body does to protect itself is to produce more mucus. However, this additional layer of mucus can interfere with your digestion. It reduces your intake of fats and fat-soluble vitamins, such as vitamin A and vitamin E, leaving you malnourished.

Our modern-day transportation networks are so sophisticated, we can eat fresh food from anywhere in the world within an 18 hour window. Food that has been grown, fertilised, and even prepared in Third World countries. Food that may be contaminated.

As gross as parasites are, we have to acknowledge that they are immensely sophisticated in their ability to conceal their presence. Many do not give any immediately identifiable symptoms. You just get a steady general degradation in your health. Your doctor then helps you to mask the symptoms with modern medicine, which does not address the root cause.

You would perhaps be horrified to realise that as much as a third of your faeces could actually be worm faeces! Experts estimate that over 160 million Americans currently have undiagnosed worm infestations.

"It is well documented that parasites will cause malnutrition by using the nutrients a victim consumes - making them unavailable for the infected person. It makes sense to use a safe reliable parasite cleanse in any chronic health challenge to ensure that you are not feeding someone else instead of yourself." - Dr. Ross Andersen, N.D.

I have deliberately left photographs out of this section, but if you aren't squeamish, I dare you to go to YouTube.com and search for "intestinal worms".

The best news about this issue is that you can easily eliminate worms from your entire body with entirely natural organic herbs that have been used for centuries. Pharmaceutical solutions tend to target specific species of parasite and do not act across a broad spectrum.

The parasite cleansing product I recommend contains a host of natural ingredients that are hostile to parasites but safe for you. They not only kill the adults, but they also kill the eggs too. They include Green Black Walnut (Hull), Clove (Flower), Pumpkin (Seed), Gentian (Root), Hyssop (Leaf), Cumin (Seed), Cramp (Bark), Peppermint (Leaf), Chinese Rhubarb (Root), Thyme (Leaf), Oregano (Leaf), and Fennel (Seed).

For more information, visit:

http://www.CancerUncensored.com/recommended-products

If you source your own anti-parasitic or colon cleansing products, just be careful to avoid products with wormwood in them. Many supplements contain wormwood, Black Walnut hulls and cloves, but wormwood has been shown to occasionally have side-effects which can include neurological damage. You are perhaps better off with worms than damage to your central nervous system!

The natural ingredients I have listed serve the same function, but without any of the risk.

A one-month course of capsules or tincture is under $40, or around £25. Repeating every few months will keep you parasite free.

Dr Hulda Clark, (1928 - 2009), is perhaps the most famous, (and controversial), advocate of parasite cleanses. She firmly believed that cancer was triggered by parasitic infection.

Whilst her opinions received mixed reactions, it stands to reason that if your body is subjected to a continuous allergic response, if your immune system is being subtly compromised, if toxins are being secreted into your tissues, and if your body is less able to absorb nutrition, then your health must be affected.

I do not believe that you can lay the cause of cancer on any one particular factor, but cleansing your system of parasites will certainly have positive health benefits. This is perhaps even more important for those who have already been diagnosed with cancer. Your body's natural processes have clearly been disrupted by something. Could this be it?

If coeliac disease and bowel inflammation has been shown in studies to significantly increase your risk of premature death, surely persistent irritation caused by parasites could fall into the same category.

There are literally hundreds of testimonials for parasite cleanses across the Internet, detailing dramatic improvements in health and quite graphic descriptions of what was eliminated from their bodies. I have added this to my own regime.

Sunbeds and Fake Tan

A study, published in the British Medical Journal in July 2012, evaluated the findings of 27 previous studies related to the use of sunbeds.

The study found that the use of sunbeds before the age of 35 was associated with an 87% increased risk of melanoma, the most dangerous form of skin cancer. A person's risk of melanoma from sunbed usage increased by 1.8% for every single sunbed session per year. The study concluded that "the cancerous damage associated with sunbed use is substantial and could be avoided by strict regulations."

The authors of the study estimated that just under 6% of malignant melanomas are due to sunbed usage, which, to be fair, is low when compared with how many skin cancers are caused by inappropriate and excessive exposure to the sun.

Sunbeds were classified by the International Agency for Research in Cancer (IARC) as 'Group 1 carcinogens' in 2009, but just like the cigarette industry, there are still customers willing to pay for it.

But many more people are aware of the cancer risk, along with premature skin ageing, so they increasingly turn to fake tan as a "safe" alternative.

Unfortunately, a primary ingredient in many spray tan products, Dihydroxyacetone, (or DHA), which turns your skin brown, has been shown in more than 10 recent laboratory studies to have risks to human health including causing damage to your DNA and potential birth defects. Some people even have an immediate allergic reaction to it.

According to Dr. Rey Panettieri, a lung specialist and toxicologist at the University of Pennsylvania, "these compounds in some cells could actually promote the development of cancers or malignancies."

DHA is approved by the US Food And Drug Administration for external use only, which means that it should not be inhaled, used near the eyes, eaten, or put on the lips. In many tanning booths, there is a significant risk of people inhaling or ingesting DHA.

So what is the solution? Well, sun exposure at moderate levels enables your body to produce vitamin D3, which has excellent anti-cancer properties and is a powerful antioxidant. Visit the Anticancer Activities section of this book to learn more about the benefits of seeking out moderate sun exposure.

But unless you do this regularly, you will not build up the Hollywood glow that many people are looking for. Equally, where do you draw the line between moderate exposure and excessive exposure?

Fortunately, DHA-free self tanning and bronzing products do exist. For example, Melvita Prosun Gradual Self-Tanning Moisturizing Gel-Cream.

However, rather than listing products which may become obsolete or discontinued over time, it is better for you to visit the following page for up-to-date brand recommendations:

http://www.CancerUncensored.com/recommended-products

Pesticides and herbicides

The full extent of the toxicity of herbicides and pesticides in food is not fully understood. From animal studies, we know that certain pesticides can cause genetic damage, fertility issues, allergy responses and cancer, so we do not want to come into contact with them, particularly within our food!

Many studies have indicated that even small doses of pesticides can have a detrimental effect on your health. Unfortunately, we live in a world where the use of pesticides and herbicides is commonplace.

Of course, your primary strategy should be to avoid pesticides in the first place. Buying organic fruit or vegetables will significantly help with this.

However, this is not always possible, nor financially practical, so the next step is to understand which fruit and vegetables are more likely to be contaminated, and how you can limit your exposure.

Based upon data from over 42,000 tests for pesticides, conducted by the US Department of Agriculture and the Food and Drug Administration (between 2000 and 2005), the following fruit and vegetables were found to contain the most pesticide residues:

- Peaches
- Apples
- Sweet bell peppers
- Celery
- Nectarines
- Strawberries
- Cherries
- Pears
- Grapes (imported)
- Spinach
- Lettuce
- Potatoes

The foods that contained the least pesticide residues were:

- Onions
- Avocado
- Sweet corn (frozen)
- Pineapples
- Mango
- Asparagus
- Sweet peas (frozen)
- Kiwi
- Bananas

- Cabbage
- Broccoli
- Papaya

This list is not provided so that you can entirely avoid certain vegetables or fruit, but so that you can take extra care in their preparation, or to prioritise which ones you buy organic.

If you cannot buy organic, be sure to wash all produce thoroughly, before using it. This will reduce levels of some pesticides, but it may not eliminate them entirely.

Peeling certain fruit and vegetables will make a big difference, but the downside is that key nutrients may be lost.

Any vegetable or fruit with a tough skin, such as apples, carrots, celery, etc, can be scrubbed with a brush under running water, which helps to remove much more of the residue.

Certain waxy-skinned items, such as apples or cucumbers can be peeled, because the waxy coating tends to retain more pesticides than other produce.

Any vegetables that grow with overlapping concentric outer leaves, such as lettuce, cabbage, leeks and onions, should have the outer layers peeled away and removed. Just wash the inner layers.

Bisphenol A in plastics

Bisphenol A, or BPA, is an organic compound used to make polycarbonate plastics or epoxy resins. Unfortunately, BPA can leak from materials that contain it. This means that it can contaminate the food and drink you consume.

BPA exhibits hormone-like properties, (which mimic oestrogen), which is why many experts have significant concern over its suitability to be used in food containers. This is to the extent that in the European Union, Canada and the US, BPA has been banned for use in baby bottles.

But it is difficult to limit your BPA exposure, because BPA is used in the epoxy resins that coat the inside of almost all food and beverage cans.

Therefore, even if your baby's bottle is BPA-free, the powdered formula you put into it is already contaminated from the can it came in - making the ban of BPA in baby bottles purely a token gesture.

A 2011 study, investigating the number of chemicals pregnant women are exposed to in the US, found BPA in 96% of the women tested.

There is currently no requirement to label BPA used in plastics. However, you can get some idea of the material used, by looking at the recycling logos on the packaging.

Generally, plastics are identified by one of 7 different Resin Identification Codes. Classes 3 and 7 may contain BPA. See an example below. This is a class 7 logo:

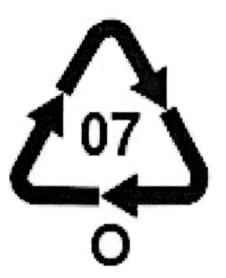

So avoid food packaging in classes 3 and 7.

Better all-round to eat fresh and avoid food and soft drinks in cans. Because even minute levels of exposure have an effect on us.

In a US report in 2008 by the National Toxicology Program, they expressed "some concern for effects on the brain, behavior, and prostate gland in fetuses, infants, and children at current human exposures to bisphenol A".

BPA has been linked in numerous studies to obesity, neurological issues, reduced thyroid function, fertility problems, intestinal permeability and inflammation, reduced immune function, and increased cancer risk (particularly in the case of breast cancer, neuroblastoma, meningioma and prostate cancer).

A 2008 study, published in the Journal of the American Medical Association, showed the results of studying 1500 people assessed for their exposure to bisphenol A. The study showed that higher levels of bisphenol A were significantly associated with heart disease, diabetes and abnormally high levels of certain liver enzymes.

Further studies conducted by the same researchers, published in January 2010, showed that patients with the highest levels of BPA in their urine samples carried a 33% increased risk of coronary heart disease.

A study conducted by the University of Texas School of Public Health in 2010, found BPA in 63 of 105 samples of fresh and canned foods, foods sold in plastic packaging, and in cat and dog foods in cans and plastic packaging. This included fresh turkey, canned green beans and canned infant formula.

A 2011 study, published in Environmental Health Perspectives, showed the contrast between eating canned / pre-packaged foods versus eating fresh. After just 3 days of eating fresh food, BPA in participants' urine decreased by 50% to 70%.

Consumer groups suggest that if you would like to lower your exposure to bisphenol A, you should avoid canned food and drink, and products supplied and polycarbonate plastic containers, (which share resin identification code 7 with many other plastics). Some packaging may indicate that the plastic is bisphenol A-free.

To avoid the possibility of BPA leaching into food or drink, the National Toxicology Panel recommends avoiding microwaving food in plastic containers, putting plastics in the dishwasher, or using harsh detergents.

Toxins we cannot avoid

In 2004, the Environmental Working Group, (EWG), took a blood sample from 10 Americans. They sent the blood samples to a laboratory to be tested for 413 different toxic chemical pollutants and industrial chemicals.

The results that came back were shocking. They discovered 287 different toxic chemicals, with an average of over 200 in each blood sample.

By category, there were 28 different waste byproducts (for example, dioxins), there were 47 different consumer product ingredients, (for example, flame retardants), and there were 212 industrial chemicals and pesticides that had been banned more than 30 years ago.

How is this possible? This is possible because the blood samples came from the umbilical cords of unborn babies. They were being supplied these chemicals in the blood of their mothers, before they were even born. It appears that the placenta does not filter these out, as previously supposed.

Of the substances detected, 134 of them caused cancer in lab studies or in people, 151 cause birth defects, 154 disrupt hormones, 186 cause infertility, 130 cause immune system toxicity and 158 of them are neurotoxic.

"The combined evidence suggests that neurodevelopmental disorders caused by industrial chemicals has created a silent pandemic in modern society". Lancet, November 8, 2006.

The experts from the chemical industries state that the pollution they create isn't a problem because it can only be measured in parts per billion once it is in the environment. This sounds very reasonable, but when you realise that even the medicines we take can be active at the parts per billion level, it is not so reassuring.

For example, Albuterol, used to reverse an asthma attack is functional at 4 parts per billion. Paxil and Cialis work at 30 parts per billion, and Nuvaring (a common birth control drug that is almost 100% effective) works at an astonishing 0.035 parts per billion.

So even minute levels of exposure matters.

Unfortunately, the environmental contamination of these toxins and pollutants is so extensive, that it is very difficult to avoid them in the air, water and food we eat. The only thing I can suggest is to ensure you use a water filter (presumably one that is free from bisphenol A!).

Long-term, it is important that we apply pressure to our politicians to clamp down on industrial pollution, because this is an issue that will accumulate for our children and grandchildren and cannot be easily reversed.

Cancer Survival Psychology

"Health and cheerfulness naturally beget each other." - Joseph Addison

Whilst there has been relatively little research conducted on the impact of psychology and cancer, there is a definite connection between mind and body that can be influenced by your levels of laughter, loneliness, depression, socialising and even placebos. This goes towards illustrating how important the mind can be in promoting health and healing. So much so, that we should not take it for granted.

"To insure good health: eat lightly, breathe deeply, live moderately, cultivate cheerfulness, and maintain an interest in life." - William Londen

Is survival a state of mind?

A study from Ben-Gurion University of the Negev, Israel, examined 255 women with breast cancer and 367 healthy women acting as controls. The researchers questioned the participants on how happy, optimistic, depressed or anxious they were before being diagnosed with breast cancer.

Researchers discovered that anxiety or depression relating to a stressful event such as divorce or bereavement appeared to be a significant contributor to the increased incidence of breast cancer. Positive states of mind, such as general happiness, played a protective role.

Is laughter the best medicine?

"A merry heart doeth good like a medicine, but a broken spirit dries the bones.." - Proverbs 17:22

Amazingly, the mechanical action of laughing has been shown to release endorphins, the body's natural pain killers. There are numerous scientific studies on the topic, including one study published in the Proceedings of the Royal Society B: Biological Sciences, which showed that being in a social group with a general sense of well-being did not trigger the same endorphins response as the physical act of laughter.

This study, showed that pain thresholds were noticeably increased during laughter. Dr Dunbar, the evolutionary psychologist at Oxford University says that it is the relaxed and contagious group laughter that is so effective. He believes that it is a form of "grooming at a distance" that fosters closeness in a group. This is very reminiscent of the grooming and delousing that maintains bonds between primates.

In fact, Dr Dunbar says that primates also engage in laughter during play. In their case, it is more a heavy panting rather than an active "ha ha".

Laughter has also been shown to:

- Lower blood pressure and LDL (bad) cholesterol.
- Increase your vascular bloodflow, (resulting in oxygenation of the blood).
- Reduce stress hormones, (such as cortisol and adrenaline).
- Exercise the diaphragm and a range of abdominal and respiratory muscles.
- Increase defence against respiratory infections, even decreasing the frequency of colds (by increasing immunoglobulin levels in saliva).
- Increase the response of your immune system, (increasing levels of gamma interferon and the action of T cells).
- Improve memory, alertness, creativity and learning, (a study at John Hopkins University Medical School, showed that humour during instruction resulted in increased test scores).

Dr Berk, a Californian physician and researcher who has studied the numerous effects of laughter explained "The ultimate reality of this research is that laughter causes a wide variety of modulation, and that the body's response to repetitive laughter is similar to the effect of repetitive exercise. The value of the research is that it may provide healthcare providers with new insights and understandings, and thus further potential options for patients who cannot use physical activity to normalise or enhance their appetite."

Dr Berk's prior work was able to demonstrate that laughter not only improves mood and reduces stress, but that is also activates the cells in the immune system that help fight cancer.

A study conducted at the Indiana State University Sycamore Nursing Centre used blood samples before and after comedy videos to demonstrate a significant increase in the numbers of natural killer cells (NK cells), which are a vital part of your immune system in the fight against cancer.

The participants were asked to complete a humour questionnaire following the videos, and the greater the level of "mirthful" laughter, the higher the immune response. The participants in the laughter group showed significantly higher levels of natural killer cells than the control group.

Just 10 minutes of laughter can also highly oxygenate our blood and organs. Two-time Nobel Prize winner Dr Otto Warburg has shown a strong connection between oxygen in the cells and good health.

A number of cancer centres are pursuing alternative therapies designed to reduce stress and increase laughter. Based upon the above research, this appears to be an excellent idea. I would advocate taking the time to engage in group laughter whether you are healthy or not. Book tickets for the next comedy gig at your local theatre, or else rent or buy comedy DVDs.

Support and relationships

"The 'I' in illness is isolation, and the crucial letters in wellness are 'we'" - Author Unknown

Having a solid support network around you can make a significant difference if you have been diagnosed with cancer. A recent study of over 440,000 Norwegian men and women, relating to 13 different types of cancer, highlighted a very interesting trend.

They discovered that men who had never married were 35% more likely to die from cancer than married men. Women who had never married were 22% more likely to die of cancer than those who were married. The most vulnerable group were unmarried men, who presumably had a smaller support network.

A similar study conducted by the University of Maryland followed patients with lung cancer. They discovered that 33% of married patients were still alive after three years, compared with just 10% of single patients. That is a three-fold increase in survival rate. Married women had the greatest three-year survival rate (46%), whilst single men had the lowest, at just 3%.

The most recent research, published in the journal Breast Cancer Research and Treatment in 2012, followed 2264 women diagnosed with early-stage invasive breast cancer, between 1997 and 2000. The study showed that socially isolated women were 34% more likely to die of breast cancer and other causes than other women who had closer social ties. The research discovered that it wasn't necessarily the quantity of social ties, but the quality.

It has been suggested that having the emotional support structure increased the chance of survival, but I would also suggest that being married or having very close relationships would also mean that the women were able to, (and encouraged to), eat better, and attend all of their hospital appointments. Consider the difference between a balanced meal prepared by a mother for her family and something a single man would eat on his own.

This research is so important, because it indicates that the impact of marriage and close relationships on cancer three-year survival rates may be greater than the impact of conventional medicine itself! So please do not neglect your emotional well-being.

Of course, that does not mean you can replace your Doctor with a spouse, but it does highlight the vital importance of a loving support network. We must consider the whole picture and not neglect the less tangible factors.

Socialising

As you will perhaps recall, from the Socialising section within the Anticancer Activities portion of this book, having a well-rounded social life actually seems to prolong your life!

Dr Lisa Berkman, of the Harvard School of Health Sciences, reported the results of a nine-year study of 7000 people aged 35 to 65. She observed that people who lacked social and community ties were almost 3 times more likely to die of medical illness than those with more extensive contacts. This was independent from socio-economic status and health practices, such as smoking, alcohol consumption, obesity and physical activity.

These findings were reinforced by a study undertaken by the California Department of Health Services, Environmental Epidemiology Section, Emeryville. 6,848 adults were studied over a 17 year period, adjusting for age, smoking, physical health at baseline, alcohol consumption, and adjusted household income. The researchers discovered that "women who were socially isolated were at significantly elevated risk of dying of cancer of all sites and of smoking-related cancers. Social connections were not prospectively associated with cancer incidence or mortality among men, but men with few social connections showed significantly poorer cancer survival rates."

In a paper published in the journal Biologist, and subsequent article in the Daily Mail, psychologist Dr Aric Sigman highlighted that the reliance on social networking sites, such as Facebook, instead of face-to-face contact could be detrimental to health.

Dr Sigman mentioned that the number of hours of face-to-face social contact has dropped substantially since 1987, as online media gradually increased.

The issue is that we already have knowledge of 209 different genes in our DNA that are "socially regulated", including genes that relate to immune response, stress responses and bonding.

For example, the bonding or "cuddle" hormone oxytocin raises and lowers, depending upon levels of close contact. Digital interaction does not influence it. If this one hormone can be moderated so dramatically by our social activity, what other genes can be switched on or off without our knowledge?

We know so little about how all of our DNA is expressed, that we could inadvertently be depriving ourselves, (or even doing harm), by physical isolation, even if we are digitally maxed out.

Dr Sigman explained that "In less than two decades, the number of people saying there is no one with whom they discuss important matters nearly tripled." "Parents spend less time with their children than they did only a decade ago. Britain has the lowest proportion of children in all of Europe who eat with their parents at the table. The proportion of people who work at home alone continues to rise."

None of this research has quantified whether it was the reduction in social interaction, or whether it was the feeling of loneliness that correlated to the increased risk, so that is currently unclear.

The message from this is to hold on to family time and to be sociable wherever you get the opportunity. Keep a slot open for family meal times, and encourage discussion. Better yet, have a family meal, and then go for a walk together.

Of course, there are never enough hours in the day, but even doing this once per week is better than never.

The placebo effect

The mind is an extraordinary thing and has the potential to influence the body in ways that current medical science cannot explain. For many years, the gold standard of medical research has been the double-blind, placebo-controlled clinical trial. This basically entails giving one group of patients the medication you are testing, and another group of individuals a fake or dummy pill which has no active ingredients. This is quite often just a sugar pill.

Such placebo trials are conducted in such a way that neither the doctors, nor the patients, know which pill they are taking. As a direct result of this approach, scientists have discovered something remarkable. Between 30% and 60% of the time, the placebo works just as well as the medication they are testing. The only variable is the person's mind and what they **believe** the pill will do for them.

In his book, The Psychobiology of Mind-Body Healing, Ernest Lawrence Rossi explains that a "Placebo's effectiveness is in proportion to what the doctor and the patient think they are using. Two placebo pills are better than one and an injection always seems to be more effective than a pill. Placebo capsules are more effective than tablets. When placebos are administered, the yellow and orange are great for mood manipulators, the dark red as a sedative; white as pain killers and lavender as hallucinogens."

At this point, you may be doubting how extraordinary the effect of the placebo can be. Allow me to share with you some of the incredible statistics obtained from medical literature and referenced in Rossi's book.

"In nine double-blind studies comparing placebos to aspirin, placebos proved to be 54 percent as effective as the actual analgesic. From this, one might expect that placebos would be even less effective when compared to a much stronger painkiller such as morphine, but this is not the case. In six double-blind studies placebos were found to be 56 percent as effective as morphine in relieving pain."

"In a recent study of a new kind of chemotherapy, 30 percent of the individuals in the control group, the group given placebos, lost their hair."

"In a study of a tranquilizer called mephenesin, researchers found that 10-20 percent of the test subjects experienced negative side effects – including nausea, itchy rash, and heart palpitations – regardless of whether they were given the actual drug or a placebo."

The extraordinary effects of placebos are "also found in double-blind studies of non-pharmacolgical insomnia treatment techniques (58% from 14 studies) and psychotropic drugs for the treatment of depression such as tricyclics (59% from 93 studies reviewed by Morris & Beck, 1974) and lithium (62% from 13 studies reviewed in Marini, Sheard, Bridges and Wagner, 1976). Thus, it appears that placebo is about 55-60% as effective as active medications irrespective of the potency of these active medications."

"In a study of morphine, there was a 50% pain reduction in 75% of the patients treated. The placebo group had a 50% pain reduction in 36% of the patients."

"In 1980 there were over 1000 articles dealing with placebos. Placebos had a high rate of activity in the areas of cough, mood swings, diabetes, anxiety, asthma, sarcoma, dermatitis, headaches, rheumatoid arthritis, radiation sickness, Multiple Sclerosis and Parkinson's."

"A group of patients were told they were given LSD when in fact they were given the placebo. They had all the physiological effects noted with LSD."

"Ipecac is a substance know to always induce vomiting. A 28-year-old female who was suffering from two straight days of nausea and vomiting was given 10cc of Ipecac syrup and told it was a new drug that stopped vomiting. In twenty minutes the vomiting had stopped completely. Her stomach showed normal contractive activity."

"During a study for headache, 120 out of 199 patients receiving the placebo obtained relief. In a test of Clofibrate versus placebo for cholesterol level and cardiovascular mortality, the placebo outperformed the drug."

"In a back pain sham therapy of four years, 40% of the placebo group improved."

"In a sham tooth-grinding surgical procedure, there was a 64% total symptom remission."

"Doctors Seidel and Abrams found that a hypodermic of saline was as effective as vaccines for chronic rheumatoid arthritis."

And so the list goes on! This data is very interesting on an intellectual level, but how can we apply it?

Perhaps the best way is to have an unwavering belief in the ability of a healthy balanced diet and exercise to help prevent cancer. If you have already been diagnosed with cancer, applying the same staunch belief that the treatment will be effective is likely to increase its effectiveness through the power of belief. Hypnotherapy may also be productive toward this end because the belief must be right to your core for it to be maximally effective.

Emotional stress and depression

Emotional stress triggers a whole cascade of biological reactions. When the brain detects a problem or a threat, a response begins in the amygdala, the hypothalamus and the pituitary gland.

This sends chemical messages to the adrenal glands to produce adrenaline and a range of glucocorticoids including cortisol. This triggers your heart to beat more quickly, for your muscles to become more tense and for your senses to sharpen. Digestion is also shut down or greatly reduced. This is known as your "flight or fight" response.

Unfortunately, glucocorticoids don't simply disappear, but in fact can remain at elevated levels for a substantial period of time. This gives you a persistent low level of chemical stress in the body, resulting in elevated blood sugar levels, a weakened immune system, the hardening of arteries, impact upon your memory and even a loss of bone mass, because cortisol blocks oestrogen receptors in your bone cells and lowers the uptake of calcium.

Stress also triggers the production of free radicals, which can increase your risk of cancer.

This mechanism has served us well throughout our history, however it is not sophisticated enough to tell the difference between a life-threatening situation and the pressure of meeting a tight deadline at work. As a result, unimportant things could be affecting your longevity.

It is very important for you to maintain a good perspective on what is really important in life, and to try to remain relaxed when you can. Stress relieving activities like yoga, can help you decompress and reduce your stress hormone levels outside of work.

Stress is a factor that you can deal with by managing your emotional states better, actively reducing stress during your time away from work, and by seeking to remove yourself from stressful situations, (perhaps by changing jobs). But other emotional factors such as depression may not be so simple.

Every year 30,000 people commit suicide in the USA alone, with the vast majority being attributed to depression. In fact, 12 million people in the US are on prescription antidepressants. People with depression frequently have a lower blood oxygen level, (by as much as 30% less), and often have an increase in cytokines, which relate to an increase in inflammation within the body. Both of these scenarios can promote the risk of cancer.

Studies also show that depression can increase your risk of heart attack by up to 6 times.

Ensuring your diet contains plenty of the amino acid tryptophan, (found in avocados), and Omega-3 essential fatty acids, (found in fish and eggs), is a good way to give your brain the raw building blocks it needs to maintain health. Of course, this is no guarantee that you can prevent or reverse depression purely with diet, but it is a good start.

A good step may be to have any mercury fillings removed, as there is a link between mercury toxicity and depression.

Both exercise and deep breathing have been shown to reduce depression and levels of the stress hormone cortisol. Laughter is likely to have a similar effect. One study of 10,000 people with high levels of cortisol demonstrated that lying down for a week only reduced their cortisol levels by 5%, whereas those who engaged in their first-ever yoga class had their cortisol levels drop by 25% within just 24 hours, and a total 65% within one month.

Taking care of your body through nutrition and exercise will certainly help with your state of mind, but sometimes there is a specific circumstantial factor at play. If something is making you unhappy, taking active steps toward resolving the situation can make all the difference and let you out from underneath the burden of it.

Life is too short to be miserable, and feeling miserable makes your life even shorter. So if this affects you, **take action** but do not rely on the answer being within a pill from your Doctor.

Unresolved emotional issues and suppressed emotions

According to www.altmd.com, "German cancer surgeon Dr. Ryke-Geerd Hamer examined thousands of cancer patients with all types of cancer. Dr. Hamer noticed that all his patients seemed to have something in common: there had been some kind of psycho-emotional conflict prior to the onset of their cancer - usually a few years before - a conflict that had never fully resolved. Dr. Hamer started including psychotherapy as an important part of the healing process and found that when the specific conflict was resolved, the cancer immediately stopped growing at a cellular level. Dr. Hamer believes that cancer-prone individuals are unable to adequately share their thoughts, emotions, fears and joys with other people. He calls this 'psycho-emotional isolation'. These people tend to hide their sadness and grief behind a brave face, appear pleasant, and avoid open conflict. According to Dr. Hamer, some people are not even aware of their emotions, and are therefore not only isolated from other people, but also from themselves."

These findings are supported by a study published in the Journal of Psychosomatic Research, which stated that "Extreme suppression of anger was the most commonly identified characteristic of 160 breast cancer patients who were given a detailed psychological interview and self-administered questionnaire. Repressing anger magnified exposure to physiological stress, thereby increasing the risk of cancer".

In Cancer Nursing, an International Journal, they explained that "Extremely low anger scores have been noted in numerous studies of patients with cancer. Such low scores suggest suppression, repression, or restraint of anger. There is evidence to show that suppressed anger can be a precursor to the development of cancer, and also a factor in its progression after diagnosis."

According to the Journal of the American Medical Association, "A 1979 study comparing long-term survivors of breast cancer with those who did not survive, scientists at John Hopkins University found that long-term survivors expressed much higher levels of anxiety, hostility and other negative emotions. Patients who were able to express their feelings lived longer than those who had difficulty in doing so."

In a study conducted at the University of Colorado in the US, researchers found that people who repressed their emotions after a traumatic event had lowered immune systems compared with those who shared their feelings. "Our work suggests that emotional disclosure may influence immune responsiveness as well as having general health benefits. We are investigating the effects of emotional expression in women with breast cancer."

Finally, researchers at Ohio State University found that highly stressed women had lower levels of natural killer cells than women who reported less stress.

"Natural killer cells have an extremely important function with regard to cancer because they are capable of detecting and killing cancer cells. Psychological interventions, such as forgiveness, have important roles in reducing stress and improving quality of life, but also in extending survival." - Barbara Andersen, Professor of Psychology, Ohio State University.

Look for the good in cancer

In order to drive you towards success, you should focus on what you want in life, rather than focusing on what you do not want. It is exactly the same with cancer. You must focus on life - and the necessary steps to make your life better and more fulfilling - not on the things you are most worried about.

Equally, it is so important to look for the positive in everything.

Many people who have survived cancer have expressed how cancer was a turning point in their lives, making them appreciate every day, helping them to find meaning in their relationships, and focus on what is important.

If cancer can help you to eat more healthily, get exercise, value relationships, learn to relax and destress, and deal with emotional baggage, then it is not entirely negative.

If you have not been diagnosed, take a moment to think about this. Can you apply the same mentality and attitudes towards your life right now? We shouldn't need a life changing health issue to focus us back onto what truly matters.

Live for today, learn to forgive, and appreciate all of the joys this wonderful world can bring. It is time to participate in life with passion and joy!

Early Detection

The National Cancer Intelligence Network (NCIN) recently announced that 24% of people who are diagnosed with cancer in the UK are only diagnosed as a result of a visit to accident and emergency wards. In patients aged 70 or over, 31% of cancer diagnosis happen via emergency admission.

The research, published in the British Journal of Cancer, examined more than 730,000 cancer patients between 2006 and 2008.

This really illustrates the weaknesses we currently have in early detection.

Clearly, prevention is where our efforts can be most effectively focused, as 85% of cancers are preventable, but early diagnosis comes a very close second, when it comes to improving outcomes.

Numerous studies indicate that early detection dramatically improves the success rate of treatment. So whilst the natural inclination is to "bury your head in the sand" and ignore the issue, this is not in your best interests.

There are a range of different kinds of diagnostic testing for cancer, ranging from chemical tests, to physical examination, to medical imaging equipment. The first we shall cover is self-examination.

Look for any changes in your health

It is important to seek medical advice if you notice any persistent changes in your health. If you ignore the symptoms and it turns out to be cancer, the delay could mean that the cancer has spread and become less easy to treat.

Every cancer has its own signs and symptoms, but these are the most important to look out for:

- A lump anywhere in your body, e.g. breast or testicle.
- A change in a skin mole.
- A sore that does not heal.
- A persistent cough or hoarseness.
- Persistent indigestion or difficulty swallowing.
- Coughing up or vomiting blood.
- Change in normal bowel habit, such as persistent diarrhoea or constipation.
- Any bleeding in the urine or bowel motions and any abnormal vaginal bleeding.
- Unexplained weight loss.
- Unexplained loss of appetite.

Having one of these symptoms does not necessarily mean that you have cancer, but you should see your doctor immediately so that the situation can be fully assessed.

There are a number of self-examinations you should conduct on a monthly basis. These can include breast examinations for women, testicular examinations for men and skin examinations for everyone - particularly if you have a higher than normal exposure to the sun.

Self-examinations:

Testicular self-examination:

Testicular cancer most commonly occurs in men aged between 15 and 34 and is one of the most common tumours seen in men under 40. If detected and treated in its early stages, testicular cancer treatment is nearly 100% successful. Unfortunately, cancerous lumps are often not discovered until the tumour is at an advanced stage. A monthly testicular self-examination can help detect lumps early in their most treatable stages.

Self-examination takes only a few minutes and is easy to do. Most lumps are not cancerous, but any lump should be checked immediately by your doctor.

The best time to check yourself is in the shower or after a warm bath. Fingers glide over soapy skin making it easier to concentrate on the texture underneath. The heat causes the skin to relax making the examination easier.

1.   Support the testicles in one hand and feel each with the other hand.
2.   Gently roll each testicle between the thumb and the fingers. You'll feel a smooth, tubular structure (epididymis) that covers the front, back and bottom of each testicle. Gently separate this tube from the testicle with your finger to examine the testicle itself.
3.   Feel for any swelling or lumps.
4.   If you detect swelling or any lumps, see a doctor without delay.

Look out for:

- Any change in size or weight of your testicles.
- A dull ache in the scrotum, groin or lower back.
- A sore, or a small patch on the shaft or tip of your penis that irritates or won't heal.

Breast self-examination:

Most breast problems present a palpable abnormality. Early detection leads to early investigation and treatment, and for this reason it is good to be in the habit of self-examination on a regular basis. Women of all ages should perform self-examination since breast problems can occur at any age.

The best time of the month to perform self-examination of the breast is after menstruation, when the breast tissue is softer and lumps are more likely to be felt. Immediately prior to menstruation the breast becomes naturally lumpy and often tender - features that can disguise a problem if one is present.

For women who are post-menstrual, or who have had a hysterectomy, a suitable time should be chosen - for example the 1st day of the month. Examination more frequently than this is probably not necessary and may lead to increased anxiety.

A woman who regularly examines her breasts will get a very clear idea of her normal breast texture and consistency, and will help her to notice if something is different.

Outlined below is one method of self-examination. Individual hospitals and specialists may advise slightly different methods, but the principles are the same.

It goes without saying that if anything is found to be abnormal then it should be examined by your doctor or a breast specialist.

In front of a mirror - hands at side:

Stand in front of a mirror with your hands on your hips. Look at the breast for any of the following:

- Asymmetry
- Lumps or swellings
- Dimples
- Ulceration
- Changes in skin colour
- Nipple retraction
- Nipple discharge

Compare one side with the other.

In front of mirror - with hands up:

Repeat the above inspection of the breasts with the hands raised above the head. Remember to look at the undersurface of the breast, especially if the breast is large.
Mirror examinations should also be done looking at the breast side-on.

In the shower:

Starting with the right side. Place the right hand above your head to "spread" the breast tissue across the chest wall. Using the flat of the left hand, examine the breast in circular motions. Make sure to cover each quadrant of the breast and end by moving your hand up into the axilla (armpit). Remember part of the breast called the axillary tail extends up to the edge of the armpit.

What to feel for:

- Lumps or thickenings (may be hard or soft, big or small, or may just feel like "something different" from usual)
- Prominent one-sided lumpiness. (Usually lumpiness when present is similar on both sides)
- Swellings or lumps in the axilla (armpit)
- Areas of tenderness

Always compare sides. Once finished examining the right breast, repeat the same procedure for the other side.

Lying down on your side:

Lie down with one hand behind your head and a pillow under your shoulder. Using the other hand palpate the breast, feeling for the same features mentioned above. Once again, use circular motions with the flat of the hand and don't forget to examine the axilla (armpit).

Finally, gently squeeze the nipple to check for discharge. Repeat this procedure lying on the opposite side.

Skin self-examination:

How to perform a skin self-examination:

Finding suspicious moles or skin cancer early is the key to treating skin cancer successfully. A skin self-examination is usually the first step in detecting skin cancer. For this, you will need a full-length mirror, a hand mirror, and a brightly lit room:

Examine your body front and back in the mirror, then the right and left sides, with your arms raised.

Bend your elbows, look carefully at your forearms, the back of your upper arms, and the palms of your hands.

Look at the backs of your legs and feet, spaces between your toes, and the soles of your feet.

Examine the back of your neck and scalp with a hand mirror.

Check your back and buttocks with a hand mirror.

Become familiar with your skin and the pattern of your moles, freckles, and other marks.

Be alert to changes in the number, size, shape, and colour of pigmented areas.

When examining moles of other pigmented areas look for a change in appearance. See if the area / mole is patchy, if it has dark and light areas, an irregular border or if it itches or bleeds. If any of these signs are present, consult your doctor immediately.

Most moles are about 6mm in diameter. If a mole becomes larger than the head of a pencil, consult your doctor.

Blood tests to detect or monitor cancer

If your doctor is concerned about a particular kind of cancer, the following tumour marker blood tests are available to them:

Cancer antigen CA 15-3 - a sensitive blood test that gives an elevated result in the presence of breast cancer, which can be useful for monitoring response to treatment. Increased levels may also be found in a variety of other malignancies including colon, stomach, gall bladder, pancreas, oesophagus, liver and lung cancer. This test should not be used for initial diagnosis but may be helpful for the detection of metastases and assessment of response to treatment.

Cancer antigen CA 125 - a blood test that gives an elevated result in the presence of malignancies of the ovary, epithelial components of the fallopian tubes, endometrium and endocervix and in some cases of breast carcinoma, malignant melanoma and endometriosis. The test is perhaps of limited value for initial diagnosis but it is useful for monitoring response to treatment.

Prostate specific antigen or PSA - a blood test to help detect prostate cancer. Low levels in a patient over 50 years of age with no symptoms suggest a normal prostate. High levels suggest prostate cancer and require further investigation. Between these levels a diagnosis of prostatic hyperplasia (an enlarged prostate) is most likely but patients should be further investigated to establish the cause of the elevated level.

Carcinoembryonic antigen or CEA - a blood test that detects a substance produced by malignant tumours, particularly of the gastrointestinal tract. This test is relatively insensitive when used for early detection, but may be useful in monitoring response to treatment of established malignancies.

Cancer antigen CA 19-9 - a blood test detecting a substance found in the serum of many patients with pancreatic, gastro-intestinal and hepatobiliary cancers. Levels are also raised (but to a lesser degree) in chronic pancreatitis, cholecystitis and various types of cirrhosis of the liver.

Alpha fetoprotein or AFP - a blood test to detect a protein found in elevated levels in the presence of liver cancer, and sometimes in the presence of testicular, ovarian, stomach, or pancreatic cancer. Cirrhosis of the liver - perhaps from hepatitis, is one of the conditions that can also elevate your AFP levels.

Placental alkaline phosphatase - a blood test to detect a substance that is present in 40-65% of patients with ovarian carcinoma and in up to 10% of other cancer patients. This test can also be used to detect 40-70% of seminomas (a form of testicular cancer). Measurement of placental alkaline phosphatase may also be used for monitoring response to treatment.

For the latest up-to-date information on new diagnostic techniques, or details of laboratories able to offer these tests, please visit:

http://www.CancerUncensored.com/early-detection

and

http://www.CancerUncensored.com/laboratories

Medical imaging

As you will see from the section on CT scans, x-rays and mammograms in the Environmental Factors to Avoid section of this book, there is inherent risk with many modern-day medical imaging techniques.

On that basis, you should try to keep your exposure to anything using x-rays or radiation to a minimum.

Unfortunately, they cannot be avoided altogether because sometimes the benefits of the diagnostic technique outweigh the risks. You must simply exercise your best judgement, alongside the recommendations of your doctor.

Fortunately, some diagnostic techniques are perfectly harmless, such as thermography.

Thermography, which uses heat signatures to spot tumours is no more dangerous than somebody taking your photo. It does not use radiation, it merely picks up on the infrared heat your body is giving off.

Other diagnostic procedures

Below is a glossary of diagnostic tests which can be carried out on different parts of your body if it is suspected that you may have cancer. This list is not exhaustive, but gives you an indication of what doctors may ask you to undergo.

Abdominal fluid aspiration - A sample of fluid that has accumulated in the abdomen can be removed for investigation by the laboratory to look for any signs of cancer.

Angiogram or arteriogram - An angiogram uses an injection of dye (which shows up on x-ray) to make the blood vessels in your body visible on a series of x-rays. If there is a tumour present, this will help to determine its location and blood supply.

Barium enema - This is where an X-ray of the bowel is taken with the aid of barium - a substance which shows up clearly on the x-ray.

Barium meal / Barium swallow - This is where an X-ray of the stomach and oesophagus is taken with the aid of barium - a substance which shows up clearly on the x-ray.

Biopsy - A biopsy is the medical removal of a sample of cells that can be examined under a microscope or chemically analysed to determine if the cells are abnormal. Some forms of cancer are not suitable for biopsy, such as testicular cancer, because it can cause the cancer to spread to other parts of the body.

Bronchoscopy - This procedure involves using a narrow, flexible tube called a bronchoscope to examine the inside of the patient's lung and airways. Under local anaesthetic, the doctor may also take cell samples or biopsies.

Central nervous system tests - in the case of suspected brain tumour, your examination may include:

- Comparing the strength of your limbs,
- An eye examination.
- A facial muscle test
- Hearing tests.
- Mental exercises.
- Checking your tongue movement, ability to swallow, etc.
- Test of your reflexes.
- Testing your ability to distinguish between hot and cold, to feel pin-pricks, etc.

Cervical smear or Pap test - The smear or Pap test is a routine screening test to detect cellular changes in the cervix. It is useful as an early warning of the potential for developing cancer, but it can also detect cervical cancer early.

Colonoscopy - A process that allows your doctor to visually examine the whole length of the large bowel using a flexible tube called a colonoscope. If there are any suspect areas, your doctor can take biopsies during the procedure.

Colour doppler - A type of ultrasound that gives a colour picture, showing the blood supply to any detected lumps. This can often be used to distinguish between a malignant and a benign lump.

Colposcopy - This involves the use of a small microscope (called a colposcope) to look at any areas of the cervix that are causing concern. A solution that can show up any abnormal areas on the cervix is used to improve the effectiveness of the technique. This procedure can also allow the doctor to take a biopsy where necessary.

Cytoscopy - A small fibre-optic telescope is used to visually examine the lining of the urethra and bladder.

Dilatation and curettage (D & C) - Which involves your doctor inserting an instrument into your uterus via the cervix, (under a general anaesthetic), in order to remove samples of tissue from the inner lining of the uterus. The tissue samples can then undergo microscopic examination for any abnormalities.

Electroencephalogram (EEG) - An EEG measures the electrical activity within the brain using wires that are placed against your head using small disks held on by a conductive gel. The resulting print-out of brain waves from the EEG machine can be examined for abnormal patterns.

Endoscopy / oesophagoscopy - Using an endoscope, your doctor can examine the oesophagus for any abnormalities. During this procedure a biopsy can be taken if there are any signs of oesophageal cancer.

ERCP (endoscopic retrograde cholangio-pancreatography) - Using a flexible instrument called an endoscope that is passed through your mouth, your doctor can inject a type of dye, (that shows up clearly on x-ray), into the opening of your bile duct and the duct of your pancreas. This enables him or her to obtain an x-ray picture of the ducts that will show any blockages. If necessary, any blockages can be removed during the same procedure.

Faecal occult blood test - To detect if there is any blood in your bowel motions.

Fine needle aspiration - Where a small amount of fluid is removed so that it can be examined for cancerous cells.

Gastroscopy - After you have fasted to empty your stomach, the doctor will use a narrow flexible telescope to examine the inside of your oesophagus and stomach under local anaesthetic. The gastroscope can be used to photograph the stomach lining and, if necessary, the doctor can conduct a biopsy at the same time.

Hysteroscopy - This technique allows your doctor to obtain a biopsy from the uterus whilst visually examining the lining using a small instrument called a hysteroscope.

Intravenous urogram (IVU or IVP) - A contrast agent is injected into a vein shortly before you are x-rayed. This procedure allows you to visualise abnormalities of the urinary system, including the kidneys, ureters and bladder.

Isotope bone scan - A radioactive substance is injected into a vein and the whole body is scanned to highlight any areas of abnormal bone. Bone scans can detect cancer earlier than conventional X-rays.

Laparoscopy - A procedure whereby the doctor is able to examine the ovaries under general anaesthetic using an instrument called a laparoscope. If there appear to be any abnormalities, the doctor can also conduct a biopsy at the same time.

Laparotomy - On occasion, ovarian cancer cannot be accurately diagnosed with laparoscopy, so investigative surgery is necessary.

Magnetic resonance imaging (MRI scan) - Unlike CT scans or traditional x-rays, MRI scans do not use ionising radiation. Instead, the patient lies within a large, powerful magnet, which creates a magnetic field. MRI gives images with good contrast between different soft tissues. This makes it especially useful when imaging cancers, muscles the heart and brain.

Mediastinoscopy - This procedure is carried out under general anaesthetic, using a tube that allows the doctor to view the inside of the chest through a small incision (at the base of the neck). The doctor can check for signs of cancer and can take samples of cells from your lymph nodes. This is of value because the lymph nodes are often the first place that cancer spreads to.

Nasendoscopy - The doctor may use a nasendoscope to get a better view of the back of the mouth and throat. The nasendoscope is a narrow flexible instrument that is passed through the nose to access the throat. It can also be used to obtain a biopsy, (under local anaesthetic), from inaccessible places within the throat.

Positron emission tomography (PET) scan - This technique can help determine how active a tumour is and whether it is malignant or benign. Having received an injection of glucose, (along with a small amount of radioactive marker), you will be scanned to provide a picture of brain activity. Tumours will show up as an abnormal area on the scan.

Proctoscopy or Sigmoidoscopy - These tests are similar to colonoscopy but use different tools to examine different areas. A proctoscope is a short tube which just goes into the rectum whilst a sigmoidoscope is a longer tube which can be passed further up into the large bowel. Again, a biopsy can be taken where necessary.

Thyroid radioisotope scan - Having injected you with a very small amount of a mildly radioactive substance, (usually iodine or technetium), your doctor will inspect your neck using a gamma camera, to see if any areas of your thyroid are not absorbing the radioactive substance. Any areas that do not absorb the material in the same way as the rest are considered abnormal.

Ultrasound - Uses ultra high frequency sound waves to painlessly create an internal image of various parts of your body. Sometimes vaginal ultrasound or trans-rectal ultrasound is used to get a clearer picture of specific areas.

X-Ray - To see if there has been any spread of the cancer to other parts of the body, especially the bones.

Cancer Information

Detailed information on each individual form of cancer is perhaps beyond the scope of this book, because methods of diagnosis change over time, along with the current best practice for treatment. On that basis, a free directory of up-to-date cancer information can be found at:

http://www.CancerUncensored.com/cancer-information

The information covers details on the individual types of cancer, the likely causes, the symptoms, how it is diagnosed, and which additional tests can be carried out.

Information on the following cancers is available:

- Bladder Cancer
- Bowel Cancer
- Brain Cancer
- Breast Cancer
- Cervical Cancer
- Kidney Cancer
- Liver Cancer
- Lung Cancer
- Malignant Melanoma
- Mouth and Throat Cancer
- Oesophageal Cancer
- Ovarian Cancer
- Pancreatic Cancer
- Prostate Cancer
- Skin Cancer
- Stomach Cancer
- Testicular Cancer
- Thyroid Cancer
- Uterine Cancer

Cancer Research

"Everyone should know that most cancer research is largely a fraud and that the major cancer research organisations are derelict in their duties to the people who support them." - Linus Pauling PhD (Two-time Nobel Prize winner)

Unfortunately, despite the thousands of women going on walks and runs for cancer research, and the hundreds of millions given in donations, cancer research is largely steered by the pharmaceutical giants.

This means that many of the potential cures, early detection techniques and preventative measures do not get investigated. In many cases, they are actively suppressed. Such discoveries would undermine the three quarters of a trillion dollar annual revenue that cancer generates.

Perhaps if you realise that the average cancer patient is worth over $300,000 in revenue over their lifetime, (and that a healthy person is not), you will see the conflict-of-interest in this industry.

"Despite the general recognition that 85 per cent of all cancer is caused by environmental influences, less than 10 per cent of the (U.S.) National Cancer Institute budget is given to environmental causes. And despite the recognition that the majority of environmental causes are linked to nutrition, less than 1 per cent of the National Cancer Institute budget is devoted to nutrition studies. And even that small amount had to be forced on the Institute by a special amendment of the National Cancer Act in 1974." - Medical Historian, Hans Ruesch.

According to a paper by the Federation of European Biochemical Societies, published in Molecular Oncology 2008, (which delved into both government and private funding of cancer research globally), this blinkered approach is everywhere. For example, of the €485 million spent between 2002 and 2006 (inclusive) by the European commission, only 0.41% (not even half of one percent) related to prevention, and less than 3.5% was spent on studying risk factors.

According to the Cancer Research UK website, "Every year Cancer Research UK spends hundreds of millions of pounds on research into preventing, diagnosing and treating cancer. We are the biggest single independent funder of cancer research in Europe, supporting the work of thousands of scientists, doctors and nurses across the UK."

Intimating that they spend hundreds of millions of pounds on research into preventing cancer is unfortunate, because it simply is not true. According to the research published on their web site, years can go by without them spending a penny on it.

If you visit the Cancer Research UK website, you can search through the research that they have been funding.

http://www.cancerresearchuk.org/science/research/who-and-what-we-fund/

You can click on a few drop-down boxes to separate it by category. If you look purely at Research Type: prevention, Cancer Type: all cancer types, only 15 studies in this category have ever been funded, and these are listed from 2005 to 2012.

This is hugely disappointing, when you realise that 85% of cancer is preventable. Surely some investment in prevention would have the biggest impact upon cancer death rates in the long term.

When you look at the research they have supported, 7 out of these 15 studies relate to drugs, pharmacology and chemopreventive agents, which isn't most people's idea of prevention. The other items relate to screening for conditions that can increase your risk of cancer, such as Helicobacter pylori infection, human papillomavirus infection and Eckstein Barr virus infection. So indirectly, they would help with prevention, but the things you would expect to see them looking into, such as the primary causes of cancer, simply are not there.

In fact, according to this list of funded research, in 2004, 2005, and 2007 they only funded a single study per year in prevention (if you can call it that).

In 2006, 2008 and 2010, the sum total that Cancer Research UK appeared to have spent on prevention was zero.

"Preventing the disease benefits no one except the patient. Just as the drug industry thrives on the 'pill for every ill' mentality, so many of the leading medical charities are financially sustained by the dream of a miracle cure, just around the corner." - Dr. Robert Sharpe.

Where are the studies showing the link between diet and cancer, both in terms of prevention and improving survival rates?

Where are the studies relating to exercise?

Where are the studies relating to environmental exposure to potentially carcinogenic factors, such as genetically modified foods, pesticides, hormones and more?

According to their accounts, for the year ended march 2012, Cancer Research UK spent £129.4 million on wages...

Their staff breakdown is as follows:

- 3,808 members of staff earning up to £60,000 per year.
- 49 members of staff earning between £60,000 and £70,000 per year.
- 36 members of staff earning between £70,000 and £80,000 per year.
- 28 members of staff earning between £80,000 and £90,000 per year.

- 13 members of staff earning between £90,000 and £100,000 per year.
- 8 members of staff earning between £100,000 and £110,000 per year.
- 8 members of staff earning between £110,000 and £120,000 per year.
- 4 members of staff earning between £120,000 and £130,000 per year.
- 4 members of staff earning between £130,000 and £140,000 per year.
- 3 members of staff earning between £140,000 and £150,000 per year.
- 2 members of staff earning between £150,000 and £160,000 per year.
- 2 members of staff earning between £160,000 and £170,000 per year.
- 2 members of staff earning between £170,000 and £180,000 per year.
- 1 member of staff earning between £210,000 and £220,000 per year.

Nearly 58% of these members of staff are involved in fundraising or support services, with only 42% carrying out "charitable activities". The fundraisers spent £148.9 million raising more funds, and historically, a chunk of the charitable activities includes the purchase of buildings.

They are also sitting on a pension scheme with assets valued at £397.7 million and total assets (less current liabilities) of £251.3 million.

It is perhaps unfair to single out Cancer Research UK, because their allocation of funds is similar to many other charities, but the half billion pounds, (493 million), they raised in 2011-2012, made little or no inroads into prevention, only a small contribution towards early detection, (much of which related to ionising medical imaging equipment), and the rest was spent on further research into conventional treatments that we already know have poor success rates.

I just feel frustrated that "cancer research" is more a matter of "cancer maintenance" and barely anyone seems to notice.

Of course, by exposing their accounts and business practices in such a critical way, I risk alienating their 40,000 loyal volunteers, who have generously given of their time to help raise funds, with the purest of intentions.

Perhaps they would be less eager to help, if they knew that much of their money is put into wages, pensions, property and more fundraising.

Very few cancer charities focus on **prevention**, and fewer still look at potential treatments outside of the mainstream protocols of surgery, chemotherapy and radiotherapy.

I do not wish to advocate any particular charity in this book, because it is hard to maintain an up-to-date league-table of genuine good causes here, but I have placed a list of what I consider to be the top cancer prevention charities (based upon my research), on:

http://www.CancerUncensored.com/cancer-prevention-charities

Cancer Treatment

In many parts of the Western world, due to European directives and federal law, the only legally accepted cancer treatment protocols involve surgery, chemotherapy or radiotherapy.

"Why would a patient swallow a poison because he is ill, or take that which would make a well man sick?" - L.F Kebler, M.D.

Does this mean that these are the only ways of treating cancer? No. But to offer anything else, your Doctor would risk losing their medical license, substantial fines and in the US, even a prison sentence.

In the late 1970s, after studying the policies, activities, and assets of the major U.S. cancer institutions, investigative reporters Robert Houston and Gary Null concluded that these institutions had become self-perpetuating organisations whose survival depended on the state of no cure.

They wrote, "a solution to cancer would mean the termination of research programs, the obsolescence of skills, the end of dreams of personal glory, triumph over cancer would dry up contributions to self-perpetuating charities and cut off funding from Congress, it would mortally threaten the present clinical establishments by rendering obsolete the expensive surgical, radiological and chemotherapeutic treatments in which so much money, training and equipment is invested. Such fear, however unconscious, may result in resistance and hostility to alternative approaches in proportion as they are therapeutically promising. The new therapy must be disbelieved, denied, discouraged and disallowed at all costs, regardless of actual testing results, and preferably without any testing at all. As we shall see, this pattern has in actuality occurred repeatedly, and almost consistently."

Indeed, many people around the world consider that they have been "cured" by therapies which have been "blacklisted" by the major cancer institutions and the medical community at large.

The individual Doctors are not necessarily to blame, but the system has overridden good conscience and common sense.

According to Dr Fereydoon Batmanghelidj, M.D, "we, as doctors, are really 007 agents of the pharmaceutical industry. We are totally blind and ignorant that the pharmaceutical industry has hijacked medicine. We learn a couple of years of physiology, but as soon as we go on the clinical side we are asked to forget those and begin to learn pharmacology, in order to treat symptoms rather than understand the primary cause of the health problem".

This view is apparently shared by many Doctors, including Lorraine Day MD (former Chief Orthopaedic Surgeon, San Francisco hospital), but they are powerless to change the system. She explained, "we doctors are taught in our medical training that virtually 80% of disease has no known cause. We are not taught to treat the underlying cause of disease, we are only taught to treat the symptoms. This does not get a person well!"

Dr Fritz Schellander explained that "Every now and again there are new drugs introduced. There is a great stir – but actually it only adds a matter of weeks or months to life expectancy. Until recently there hasn't been a single study that could conclusively show that radiotherapy to the breast has any effect on survival and yet we apply it almost routinely to often very young patients. Many patients would not choose chemotherapy and radiotherapy if they knew the real facts, the real scientific evidence. A study has been reported which claims that nearly 70% of oncologists would not opt for chemotherapy, if their turn came."

Part of the way the stranglehold has been maintained is the way in which the success rate of mainstream treatments are reported.

The significant difference is between **relative** success rates and **absolute** success rates.

Firstly, let me define success rate.

In the cancer research industry, the closest thing you get to a "cure" is a five-year survival. So if you survive five years and a day, you were a "success".

Cancer is the only disease where you can die of the condition you were "successfully" treated for. It sounds ludicrous, but this has enabled the cancer industry to massage statistics.

In the same vein, early detection has increased so-called survival rates, because by detecting the disease earlier, it isn't necessarily that the patient will live longer overall, but they are more likely to survive five years from diagnosis.

What many people do not realise, is that their tumour may have taken as long as 10 years to develop to the extent where it was noticeable.

Therefore, much of the improvements in success rate of cancer treatment is down to the way the statistics are handled, as opposed to the actual effectiveness of the treatment.

The difference between relative success rates and absolute success rates is even more important.

Imagine you had a cancer treatment, where 2 more people out of every 100 people would survive five years after receiving it (as opposed to no treatment at all). If you now develop a new cancer treatment, such as a different variation of chemotherapy, if it now saves 3 additional people out of every 100, it has a relative success rate of 50%. This is because it "cures" 50% more people than the previous methodology.

However, if you were to express the data as an absolute success rate, you would say that the absolute success rate of that treatment was 3%. i.e. 3 out of every 100 people.

Just to clarify, that does not mean only 3% of the people survive, it means that 3% MORE people survive than if offered no treatment at all.

Look how much easier it is to justify putting somebody through chemotherapy and radiotherapy when you can talk about a 50% relative success rate, rather than a 3% absolute success rate of the treatment.

A study of every randomised controlled clinical trial of chemotherapy performed in the US, (from 1990 to 2004), was conducted and published under the title "The Contribution of Cytotoxic Chemotherapy to 5-year Survival in Adult Malignancies". The results showed the following cancer "cure" statistics attributable to chemotherapy - based upon absolute success rates:

Pancreas	0%
Soft Tissue Sarcoma	0%
Melanoma	0%
Uterus	0%
Prostate	0%
Bladder	0%
Kidney	0%
Unknown Primary Site	0%
Multiple Myeloma	0%
Stomach	0.7%
Colon	1%
Breast	1.4%
Head and neck	1.9%
Lung	2%
Rectum	3.4%
Brain	3.7%
Oesophagus	4.9%
Ovary	8.9%
Non-Hodgkin's Lymphoma	10.5%

Cervix	12%
Testes	37.7%
Hodgkin's Disease	40.3%

Testicular cancer and Hodgkin's disease, which both appear to be quite responsive to chemotherapy, only represent 2% of the total number of cancers.

When you strip away the relative success rates, modern chemotherapy, (which can destroy your immune system, and rob you of your quality of life without giving you any more time), leaves a lot to be desired.

"In oncology we have the problem that progress has been very, very slow and we are still living with the paradox of treating cancers with carcinogenic agents! This feels completely wrong to me! - Dr Fritz Schellander

The overall average was a 2.1% improvement in five-year survival rate compared with not using chemotherapy at all. The same process, when applied to Australian data resulted in a 2.4% improvement in five-year survival rate.

Again, just to clarify, it didn't mean that only 2.1% of Americans survived cancer, it just meant that chemotherapy only contributed to an additional 2.1% people having a five-year survival rate.

It is no wonder that the American Cancer Society stated "Surgery, radiation therapy, and chemotherapy seldom produce a cure" in their "Cancer facts and figures 2007" literature.

So 2.1% more of the US patients survived for 5 years when given chemotherapy. But for the 97.9% of patients who did not get an increase in five-year survival rate, let us look at the price they paid for the attempt - the side effects of chemotherapy and/or radiotherapy include:

Abnormal ECG's, Abdominal Cramps, Anemia, Arterial Damage, Bleeding Sores, Bleeding Ulcers, Blood Clotting, Bone Marrow Suppression, Brain Shrinking, Chromosomal Lesions, Chronic Radiation Proctitis, Constipation, Cumulative Toxicity, Cystitis, Deafness, Decreased White Cell Count, Dehydration [severe], Destroys linings of intestines, Destroys Mucous Membranes, Destroys Skin, Diarrhea [severe], Difficulty Absorbing Food, Dizziness, Endometriosis, Flu Symptoms, Gastrointestinal Bleeding, Hair Loss, Heart Disease, Hematological Problems, Hyper Sensitivity Reactions, Hypertension, Immune System Damage, Impaired Concentration, Impaired Eye Sight, Impaired Hearing, Impaired Language Skills, Impaired Memory, Impotence, Increased Infections, Joint Pain, Kidney Damage, Leucopenia, Liver Fibrosis, Liver Lesions, Loss of Appetite, Loss of Libido, Loss of Nerve Function, Loss of Taste, Lung Damage, Lymph edema, Malnutrition, Nausea, Necrosis, Neurological Damage, Neuropathy, Neutropenia, Nerve Damage, Numbness, Oral Ulcers, Permanent Disabilities, Psychological Distress, Radiation Burns, Radiation poisoning, Renal Dysfunction, Sexual Dysfunction, Soreness of Gums and Throat, Sterility, Stroke, Sudden Menopause, Suicide, Ulceration, Urinary Bleeding, Vascular Damage, Vomiting [severe], Weakness, Weight Loss, and TOXIC DEATH!

Was it really worth it? Especially when you look at Doctors such as Dr Joseph Issels in Germany, who was able to get a 24% success rate from over 16,000 cases over a 40 year period using alternative therapies, even after chemotherapy and radiotherapy had done their damage.

Or a 22% 5-year success rate for "incurable" forms of brain cancer achieved by Dr Burzynski, M.D., Ph.D. in Texas, using his revolutionary Antineoplastons treatment.

Diffuse, intrinsic, childhood brainstem glioma had never before been cured in any scientifically controlled clinical trial in the history of medicine. Now, Dr Burzynski has "cured" dozens of patients as part of his FDA approved clinical trials - trials using treatment methods outside of the mainstream Western cancer treatment protocols. This is after the FDA spent 10 years and $60 million of tax payer's money trying to shut him down!

As I mentioned in the introduction, I have pulled no punches. This data is shocking and will feel contradictory to what we have been spoonfed by the Cancer research organisations who are forever pushing the "cancer cure just around the corner" mentality, even whilst they throw more money at methodologies that have not improved survival rates for decades.

How on earth have the medical and cancer research communities been able to keep the fact that chemotherapy barely works under wraps?

Is a 2.1% improvement worth hundreds of billions of dollars in cancer research conducted over decades, when 85% of cancer is preventable in the first place? If we had focused on prevention all those years ago, most of the cancer patients would never be in the position to even need treatment.

In a recent patent application by the US government, (when they attempted to patent Dr Burzynski's antineoplastons - which were already patented!), the US government even admitted, "Current approaches to combat cancer rely primarily on the use of chemicals and radiation, which are themselves carcinogenic and may promote recurrences and the development of metastatic disease."

In a German study of elderly breast cancer patients (80 years old and older), where half received treatment involving chemotherapy and the other half received no treatment at all, the untreated group lived an average of 11 months longer.

An article on www.naturalsociety.com says it all...

"Cancer drugs, pushed by many drug companies as the only 'scientific' method of combating cancer alongside chemotherapy, have been found to actually make cancer worse and kill patients more quickly. The findings come after research was conducted on the cancer drugs at the Beth Israel Deaconess Medical Center in Boston. Sold at a premium price to cancer sufferers, it turns out these drugs are not only ineffective but highly dangerous.

Something known as anti-angiogenesis is the primary function behind many such widely-used cancer drugs that were analyzed in the study. Researchers examined drugs such as imatanib (a leukemia drug that goes by the brand name Gleevec) and sunitinib (a drug for gastrointestinal tumors — brand name Sutent), finding that these drugs may initially reduce tumor size but afterwards cause tumors to 'metastasize' aggressively. This means that the tumors come back much stronger and grow much larger than their original size.

As a result, patients develop life-threatening tumors that oftentimes kill patients more quickly as a result of taking the drug.

When study researchers induced anti-angiogenesis in mice, there was an initial 30% decrease in the volume of the tumor over 25 days. Afterwards, however, the tumors that had metastasized to the lungs tripled. Researchers published the findings in the January 17 issue of Cancer Cell, with study authors shocked by the findings.

"Whatever manipulations we're doing to tumors can inadvertently do something to increase the tumor numbers to become more metastatic, which is what kills patients at the end of the day," said study author Dr. Raghu Kalluri.

It is clear that these cancer drugs are virtually ineffective at treating cancer, even killing patients who may have otherwise survived. Of course a number of natural anti-cancer substances do exist that have been found to be largely effective in reducing tumor size and most importantly combating the onset of cancer. Perhaps the most amazing anti-cancer substance for your health is high quality turmeric. Turmeric has been found to reduce tumors by an astounding 81% in recent cancer research. And contrary to cancer drugs, turmeric does not come loaded with deadly side effects.

Quite the opposite, turmeric instead comes with beneficial properties that can prevent your risk of disease and positively affect over 560 conditions.

Vitamin D is another essential anti-cancer nutrient. Amazingly, vitamin D is much more effective than pharmaceutical drugs at fighting cancer, and is virtually a free nutrient. Instead of paying a premium price for deadly cancer drugs, your vitamin D levels can be significantly improved by soaking up some sunlight. It is important to receive a blood test to ensure you are within the optimal vitamin D level range. The correct test you should receive is 25(OH)D, also called 25-hydroxyvitamin D. The optimal range is 50-70 ng/ml, though if you are fighting cancer or heart disease it is 70-100 ng/ml."

In a further article, published on www.activistpost.com, it was highlighted that chemotherapy can make cancer far worse, due to its damaging effects on healthy surrounding tissues...

"A team of researchers looking into why cancer cells are so resilient, accidentally stumbled upon a far more important discovery. While conducting their research, the team discovered that chemotherapy actually heavily damages healthy cells and subsequently triggers them to release a protein that sustains and fuels tumor growth. Beyond that, it even makes the tumor highly resistant to future treatment.

Reporting their findings in the journal Nature Medicine, the scientists report that the findings were 'completely unexpected'. Finding evidence of significant DNA damage when examining the effects of chemotherapy on tissue derived from men with prostate cancer, the writings are a big slap in the face to mainstream medical organizations who have been pushing chemotherapy for years as the only option available to cancer patients.

The news comes after it was previously revealed by similarly breaking research that expensive cancer drugs not only fail to treat tumors, but actually make them far worse. The cancer drugs were found to make tumors 'metastasize' and grow massively in size after consumption. As a result, the drugs killed the patients more quickly.

Known as WNT16B, scientists who performed the research say that this protein created from chemo treatment boosts cancer cell survival and is the reason that chemotherapy actually ends lives more quickly.

Co-author Peter Nelson of the Fred Hutchinson Cancer Research Center in Seattle explains:

"WNT16B, when secreted, would interact with nearby tumour cells and cause them to grow, invade, and importantly, resist subsequent therapy."

The team then complemented the statement with a word of their own:

"Our results indicate that damage responses in benign cells... may directly contribute to enhanced tumour growth kinetics."

Meanwhile, dirt cheap substances like turmeric and ginger have consistently been found to effectively shrink tumors and combat the spread of cancer. In a review of 11 studies, it was found that turmeric use reduced brain tumor size by a shocking 81%. Further research has also shown that turmeric is capable of halting cancer cell growth altogether. One woman recently hit the mainstream headlines by revealing her victory against cancer with the principal spice used being turmeric.

This accidental finding reached by scientists further shows the lack of real science behind many 'old paradigm' treatments, despite what many health officials would like you to believe. The truth of the matter is that natural alternatives do not even receive nearly as much funding as pharmaceutical drugs and medical interventions because there's simply no room for profit. If everyone was using turmeric and vitamin D for cancer (better yet, cancer prevention), major drug companies would lose out."

It makes grim reading when you know that the main institutions take decades to change their strategies.
But it would be entirely irresponsible of me to recommend, or dissuade you from engaging in any particular course of treatment. It is between you and your doctor to decide what is appropriate for you, but I would ask you to question your doctor about the absolute success rate of his or her proposed course of treatment, and whether it is wise to engage in a treatment that deteriorates, if not destroys, your immune system and quality of life.

If your Doctor cannot give you accurate absolute statistics, or will not support your choices, perhaps you should find a different Doctor?

"Alternative" Medicine

"If you are in the health profession and want to get a lot of people angry at you, begin to cure incurable diseases". David J Getoff, Naturopath and Board Certified Clinical Nutritionist.

This section is too brief to do justice to any of the alternative protocols listed. However, the information presented here does serve as an excellent starting point to make you aware of the possibilities.

It also gives you a glimpse of the darker side of the medical and cancer research establishment.

As you can imagine, your doctor is highly unlikely to present you with this information, so please take the responsibility of educating yourself.

This section should be viewed as a springboard to propel you towards conducting your own research, prior to making any treatment decisions.

Of course, further up-to-date reading is always available at:

http://www.CancerUncensored.com/alternative-medicine

This section has been entitled Alternative Medicine because it is not permitted to be called "treatment" under current legislation / regulations.

This is unfortunate, because much of this medicine is based upon solid scientific principles. It just involves methodologies that are not easy to monetise, cannot be patented, or else are from outside of the mainstream "club".

As a result, mainstream medicine will criticise the level of data available, whilst simultaneously refusing to make the funding or research opportunities available to help it to become part of accepted mainstream medicine. Equally, history is always written by the victor, so do not believe everything you read!

I must reiterate that the discussion of any of these forms of alternative medicine is not an endorsement or recommendation. Some of this information is purely historical.

This section is merely a starting point for your ongoing research and consultation with your Doctor.

"Look at what went wrong, try to correct it and give an extra little push to the body. If you only aim for homeostasis then you might not get the desired effect." - Dr Etienne Callebout

What do we know about cancer?

In 1931, Dr Otto Warburg won the Nobel Prize for proving that cancer cannot survive in an alkaline, oxygen-rich environment. He showed that cancer in fact thrives in an acidic, low-oxygen environment.

We know that most individuals with cancer are deficient in a range of vitamins, minerals, essential fatty acids, fibre and enzymes. This makes it harder for a person's immune system and body to function as it should.

We know that a wide range of natural dietary compounds can also inhibit or even kill cancer cells.

We know that most individuals with cancer do less exercise and therefore spend less time with their body well oxygenated.

We know that many cancer patient's bodies are over-taxed with toxins and their body needs assistance to remove them.

We also know that cancer cells absolutely love sugar. In fact, cancer cells have been shown to have 96 sugar receptor sites, where normal healthy cells only have four! Unfortunately, a high sugar diet also lowers your body's pH, making your body more acidic and cancer-friendly.

Finally, studies have shown that many cancer patients have suffered an emotional trauma in the recent past, or have other unresolved emotional issues. Just like a persistent allergy, persistent underlying emotional stress also causes a dip in your immune system and an excess of free radicals, which could create a window for cancer to take hold.

With all of this information in mind, it makes perfect sense that avoiding cancer, or attempting to reverse its formation should involve:

- Dietary changes to help give the body the raw materials it needs, (and the compounds that cancer hates), along with helping your body to become more alkaline. The greater your fresh fruit and vegetable intake, the less meat and dairy you eat, the more alkaline your system becomes and the more electrons your food can donate to your cells and to fight free radicals.
- The more exercise you do, the greater your natural production of antioxidants, the better your lymph circulates and the longer you spend in a well oxygenated state.
- Avoiding processed sugar, artificial sweeteners, phosphates, monosodium glutamate and other food additives means that you are not inadvertently stimulating the growth of any cancer cells.
- Detoxifying your colon, kidneys, blood, liver and mouth (dental).
- Addressing your emotional health, to ensure a positive outlook and peace of mind.

This is fundamental and well-established science, which should be the starting place for all forms of prevention or "treatment".

Unfortunately, mainstream medicine is highly political and financially driven. So despite the fundamental logic behind a lot of alternative medicine, the establishment is anything but friendly towards those who undermine the current status quo.

Take a look at the work of the pioneers in this industry - who had to fight every step of the way to be heard.

Dr Krebs and Vitamin B17

As I mentioned in the Apples section of this book, Vitamin B17, otherwise known as Amygdalin or Laetrile is a nitriloside, which naturally occurs in a range of foods, including some berries, some beans, grasses, leaves, nuts, flax, bitter almonds, beansprouts, millet and certain fruit seeds. In fact it is found in over 1200 edible plants. It is particularly prevalent in the seeds of Apples, apricots and peaches.

It was originally brought to the public eye by Dr Ernst T Krebs, but was quickly squashed by the pharmaceutical industry.

Dr Krebs applied for a patent for the process of producing a metabolite form for clinical use that he called Laetrile. As part of his research, he had discovered that the Hunza people (who live in the Himalayan mountains of northern India), had levels of cancer so extraordinarily low that they were considered to be virtually cancer-free.

He discovered that they consume large quantities of millet and apricots (including the seeds), which gave them a dietary intake of vitamin B17 greater than 100 times more than the average American.

Each molecule of vitamin B17 contains one unit of hydrogen cyanide, one unit of benzaldehyde and two units of glucose tightly locked together. The cyanide molecule can only become dangerous if the entire B17 molecule is dismantled.

Fortunately, we lack the enzymes necessary to break the molecule down, which makes it harmless to healthy tissue. Cancer cells, however, contain the necessary enzyme called beta-glucosidase. That means that when vitamin B17 disperses throughout your body, it is only broken down into cyanide within cancer cells, thereby creating a targeted therapy.

However, mainstream medicine and the pharmaceutical industry do not concur with the research, which is unsurprising considering that if vitamin B17 were proven to be effective in the treatment of cancer, it would entirely undermine $200 billion per year in revenues.

Dr Ralph Moss, when interviewed on the Laura Lee Radio Show in 1994 explained...

"Twenty years ago I was hired at Memorial Sloane Kettering (MSK) Cancer Centre in New York as the science writer, later promoted to assistant director of public affairs. Shortly after I went to work there I went to visit an elderly Japanese scientist, Kanematsu Sugiura, who astonished me when he told me he was working on Laetrile (B17), at the time it was the most controversial thing in cancer ...reputed to be a cure for cancer.

We in public affairs were giving out statements that Laetrile was worthless, it was quackery, and people should not abandon proven therapies. I was astonished that our most distinguished scientist would be bothering with something like this, and I said why are you doing this if it does not work?

He took down lab books and showed me that in fact Laetrile is dramatically effective in stopping the spread of cancer. The animals were genetically programmed to get breast cancer and about 80 - 90% of them normally get spread of the cancer from the breast to the lungs which is a common route in humans, also for how people die of breast cancer, and instead when they gave the animals Laetrile by injection only 10-20% of them got lung metasteses. And these facts were verified by many people, including the pathology department."

When asked "So this is verified, that Laetrile can have this positive effect?", Moss replied,

"We were finding this and yet we in public affairs were told to issue statements to the exact opposite of what we were finding scientifically, and as the years went by I got more wrapped up in this thing and 3 years later I said all this in my own press conference, and was fired the next day, 'for failing to carry out his most basic job responsibility' - ie to lie to the public about what goes on in cancer research."

"Dr Sugiura, never renounced the results of his own studies, despite the fact they put enormous pressure on him to do so."

"When I was at MSK a lot of very weird things started to happen to me, there was this cognitive distance between what I was told, and was writing about treatment, especially chemotherapy, and what I was seeing with my own eyes.

One time I heard the head of the intensive care unit give a talk in which he bragged about how he had one of the lowest mortality rates in his unit. I went out to lunch with him, where he became a bit inebriated, and told me how he managed to get those statistics - by wheeling the dying patients out into the corridor where they died and didn't sully our departments record."

Unfortunately, it is increasingly apparent that public health, corporate finances, politics and even basic human decency cannot all be put first without something suffering.

In my honest opinion, I believe vitamin B17 is worthy of further research - to the degree that I have added apricot kernels and apple seeds to my diet. But it is likely to be just one of many tools and not the entire solution.

"The anti-cancer effect of amygdalin was demonstrated in Mexico by government sponsored research under Dr. Mario Soto De Leon and its use is legal. Dr Soto was the first medical director of the Cydel Clinic in Tijuana (taken over by Dr Manner). It is very important that it be prepared and administered correctly in sufficient dosage or it will not be effective. The trial performed at the Mayo Clinic in the early 80's involved the use of the racemic mixture rather than the levo-rotary form and thus was only 10% of the strength required. In spite of this, towards the end of the experiment, the patients began to show improvement, but it was discontinued and declared ineffectual." - from the book Deadly Deception by Dr Willner.

Dr Burzynski and Antineoplastons

Back in the early 1970s, Dr Burzynski discovered that there was a fundamental difference between the peptides in the blood and urine samples of cancer patients versus healthy individuals. The cancer patients were missing some substances that are normally present. He named these antineoplastons.

He theorised that by synthesising the missing peptides and putting them back into the body of the cancer patient, he could restore the natural balance and help the body to fight off the cancer. Dr Burzynski has been artificially synthesising these substances since the 1980s in order to help his patients, and for them to be used in clinics outside of the USA.

Dr Burzynski has worked for decades to save lives and to prove the efficacy of his treatments, despite a running battle with the FDA and the Texas State Board of Medical Examiners, who were allegedly under pressure by the FDA.

Appallingly, whilst the FDA was frittering away over $60 million of taxpayers money, the US government, via the Department of Health was simultaneously filing patents on Dr Burzynski's discoveries.

If there is no credence to Dr Burzynski's discovery, then why are so many of his patients alive years, if not decades, after diagnosis of "incurable" forms of brain cancer?

Equally, why would the US government patent application state "the neoplastic conditions treatable by this method includes neuroblastoma, acute promyelocytic leukaemia, acute myelodysplasia, acute glioma, prostate cancer, breast cancer, melanoma, non-small cell lung cancer, medulloblastoma, and Burkitt's lymphoma." (Source: US patent #5,605,930; "Compositions and Methods for Treating and Preventing Pathologies Including Cancer"; Filed 3/7/94; Approved 2/25/97 The USA Dept. of HHS.)

Incredibly, the string of 11 related patents were granted despite them being copycats of a patent that Dr Burzynski had already been granted several years before!

For more information on Dr Burzynski's discovery, and the video detailing his legal battles to bring this discovery into mainstream medicine, visit:

http://www.CancerUncensored.com/alternative-medicine

or visit Dr Burzynski's web site:

http://www.burzynskiclinic.com

Dr Issels and Issels Integrative Oncology

Born Nov. 21, 1907 - Died Feb. 11, 1998.

In a study of 370 cancer patients on Dr. Issels' programme, 87% (322) were still alive with their cancers in regression after five years.

Dr Issels is often viewed as being the "Father of integrative medicine", whereby he would use all of the tools at his disposal - from conventional protocols to alternative medicine, including Coley Vaccines and Hyperthermia treatment, (further details of these strategies follow in this section).

"This Integrative Cancer Treatment was pioneered in Germany by the renowned cancer specialist, Josef M. Issels, M.D., at the world's first hospital with 120 beds dedicated to the treatment of advanced cancers and especially those resistant to chemotherapy and other standard therapies. It has been internationally known for its remarkable complete long-term tumor remissions for over 50 years."

"Issels Integrative Oncology is a very comprehensive strategy that integrates, (with equal importance), therapies directed against the cancer cells and tumors, as well as therapies designed to restore the patient's complex immune, regulatory, and repair mechanisms to recognize and kill cancer cells.

It is always individualized and comprises integrative immunotherapy, including cancer vaccines, cytokines, cell protocols, and other state-of-the art, research-based therapies, as well as standard treatment when indicated."

http://www.issels.com

For more information on Dr Issels' methodologies and other alternative practitioners visit:

http://www.CancerUncensored.com/alternative-medicine

Dr Coley and Coley's Vaccine

"It could just be that the results achieved by Coley are the best results we will ever achieve in the treatment of cancer." - Dr Charles Starnes, Ph.D. (an immunologist).

It is well-known that we have many thousands of cancer cells in our body at any one moment in time. However, our immune system is persistently destroying the abnormal cells.

In situations where the immune system is unable to keep up with the build-up of cancer cells, this is where it is believed the condition we know and call "cancer" begins.

Dr William Coley was a surgical oncologist who discovered a way of stimulating the immune system to increase our immune response to both disease and cancer. The theory being, that if the immune system could be stimulated to greater effect by a false stimulus, it could destroy the excess cancer cells, in the same way that our bodies normally do on a daily basis.

Coley observed and recorded the relationship between infection and spontaneous cancer regression as early as 1884.

Coley's vaccine consisted of a mixture of dead bacteria from a range of different species. When administered to patients, the dead bacteria would trigger a fever and an immediate immune response.

One rationale behind the effectiveness of this process argues that macrophages, (a type of white blood cell in our immune system), are either in "repair mode", furthering the growth of cancer, or in "defense mode", destroying cancer.

Unfortunately, macrophages only operate in "defense mode" if there is some recognised enemy. As cancer tissue is not recognised as an enemy, (but as normal body tissue), there is a need to bring more macrophages into "defense mode" by simulating an infection.

The simulated infection results in a real fever. Unlike mechanically induced hyperthermia (a raising of body temperature), real fever not only means the heating up of the body but it also creates increased activity of the immune system. Therefore, a fever response is seen as a precondition for a therapy using Coley's vaccine to work.

Coley's vaccine, otherwise known as Coley's Toxin, was used to treat cancer between 1893 all the way up until 1963 in the US. Unfortunately, due to the massive thalidomide controversy and the Kefauver Harris Amendment of 1962, (otherwise known as the "Drug Efficacy Amendment" to the Federal Food, Drug, and Cosmetic Act), Coley's Toxins were assigned "new drug" status by the FDA, making it illegal to prescribe them outside of clinical trials.

In Germany, Coley's Toxins were produced by the small German pharmaceutical company, Südmedica, and sold under the trade name Vaccineurin. However, production ceased by 1990 because of a lack of re-approval by the German Federal Institute for Drugs and Medical Devices.

According to a radio interview on the Laura Lee Radio Show in 1994, with Ralph Moss, Ph.D. a science writer at Memorial Sloan-Kettering Cancer Centre in the 1970s...

"It was discovered at MSK in 1893 and the results... over a 1000 people were treated with it. It is basically a high fever treatment. Some guy rang a radio show I was on; he had a sarcoma that was operated on, it spread, and his doctor sent him to Dr Coley. He was 13 at the time and 95 now. This is 82 years. Sarcoma is an incurable disease. A blow away treatment.

In advanced terminal breast cancer they got complete remissions in 50% of the cases using this treatment. That is not saying what you would get if you used it in conjunction with surgery, you may get 100%... it is criminal. I have known about this and lived with it for 20 years.

You know what? THEY know about it at Sloane Kettering. They even put Coley's picture in their publicity material, as a pioneer of immunology, but they would never use the treatment themselves.

They want to develop DRUGS that can be spun off like Tumour Necrosis Factor, like these other immunologically based drug treatments, highly toxic, destructive of the immune system, incredibly expensive. This is really an effective treatment and it's an OUTRAGEOUS crime of the century that we at MSK were able to cure cancer a 100 years ago that they can't cure today. This is a fraud being perpetrated on the public..."

When asked, "So why isn't the New York Times writing about this?", Moss replied, "The chairman of the board of Bristol Myers, the main company producing anti-cancer drugs, who also happens to be on the board of MSK, is also on the board of the New York Times."

Five-year survival rates, based on data collected by Helen Coley Nauts, (Coley's daughter), in the 1970's, showed: 65% for patients with inoperable breast cancer; 69% for patients with inoperable ovarian cancer; and 90% for those with Osteosarcoma, (bone cancer). Soft tissue sarcoma had a five-year survival rate of 48%, and Lymphoma survival was 58%.

Research conducted at Memorial Sloane Kettering Cancer Centre in 1976 showed that patients with advanced non-Hodgkinson's lymphoma experienced a 93% remission rate versus 29% for the group that was treated with chemotherapy alone.

The cost of this process? Well material costs were virtually nil. Perhaps $10 in materials will treat many cancer patients.

The fact that the pharmaceutical giant, Pfizer, acquired the Coley Pharmaceutical Group, clearly demonstrates that there may be a place for the use of, (or suppression of), these discoveries in modern medicine.

Specialized medical doctors in Germany still apply Coley's toxins to patients today. They can do so legally because unapproved medications may be produced in Germany, although they may not be sold or given away.

Physicians can go to special laboratories and produce Coley's toxins there using their own hands. Coley's toxins may still be applied by a licensed medical doctor, because in Germany they have "Therapiefreiheit" ("therapy freedom"), the legal right to apply whichever therapy a licensed physician considers to be appropriate in the light of their medical knowledge.

For more information on Dr Coley's methodologies and other alternative practitioners visit:

http://www.CancerUncensored.com/alternative-medicine

Dr Johanna Budwig - The Budwig Diet

Dr Budwig, (30 September 1908 – 19 May 2003), was nominated seven times for the Nobel Prize. She claimed to have a greater than 90% success rate with her protocol which was used on all kinds of cancer patients over a 50 year period.

"What she (Dr. Johanna Budwig) has demonstrated to my initial disbelief, but lately, to my complete satisfaction in my practice is: CANCER IS EASILY CURABLE, the treatment is dietary/lifestyle, the response is immediate; the cancer cell is weak and vulnerable; the precise biochemical breakdown point was identified by her in 1951 and is specifically correctable, in vitro (test-tube) as well as in vivo (real)... " - Dr. Dan C. Roehm M.D. FACP (Oncologist and former cardiologist) in 1990.

Dr Budwig's protocol relied upon eliminating the four suspected "causes" of cancer:

- Nutritional deficiency.
- A weakened immune system.
- Toxins.
- Oxygen deprivation.

She did this through a diet rich in flaxseed oil, mixed with cottage cheese or quark, along with meals high in fruit, vegetables and fibre. She also advocated the avoidance of refined sugar, animal fats, meat and processed oils.

Some of Dr Budwig's most compelling research showed that refined vegetable oils, margarine and deep-fried foods, deprived the cells in your body of oxygen.

Mainstream science has already proven that the nucleus of every cell carries a positive charge, and the membrane on the outside of each cell carries a negative charge. Further research shows that the negative charge on the outside of healthy cells is three times stronger than in cancer cells.

It is believed that if the negative charge on the outside of cells is diminished, it also reduces the cell's ability to absorb oxygen and nutrients, whilst simultaneously making it much harder for the cell to excrete waste products.

Dr Budwig discovered that many types of processed oil, (which have been heated for up to an hour during processing), strip the negative charge from the surface of our cells. Dr Budwig's research showed that chemically processed fats and oils are not water-soluble when they are bound to protein in your body. They end up damaging the action of the heart, blocking circulation, inhibiting the renewal process of your cells and impeding the free flow of blood and lymphatic fluids.

Omega-3 essential fatty acids reverse this process.

On that basis, an abundance of "dead" heat treated oils and a lack of fresh omega-3 oils could be a major contributor to our current cancer crisis.

Dr Budwig was a firm advocate of cold-pressed oils, which had not undergone extensive processing. Flaxseed, olive oil, sunflower oil, virgin coconut oil and safflower oil were all recommended.

But the mainstay of her treatment, flaxseed oil combined with cottage cheese or quark was far superior. Dr Budwig found that this combination helped to restore the electrical balance of your cells and was very high in Omega-3 essential fatty acids.

As I mentioned in the "The Basics" section of this book, the average Western diet has a ratio of around 15 parts of omega-6 to 1 part omega-3.

In 2009, the Center for Genetics, Nutrition and Health in Washington DC, published study data that indirectly confirms Dr Budwig's findings and beliefs. They stated that "such a high ratio has been shown to increase the likelihood of many diseases, including cardiovascular disease, cancer, and inflammatory and autoimmune diseases, whereas increased levels of omega-3 (a low omega-6/omega-3 ratio) exert suppressive effects.

In the secondary prevention of cardiovascular disease, a ratio of 4/1 was associated with a 70% decrease in total mortality. A ratio of 2.5/1 reduced rectal cell proliferation in patients with colorectal cancer... The lower omega-6/omega-3 ratio in women with breast cancer was associated with decreased risk. A ratio of 2-3/1 suppressed inflammation in patients with rheumatoid arthritis, and a ratio of 5/1 had a beneficial effect on patients with asthma."

Dr Budwig is sadly no longer with us, however her research, books and recipes for use at home are still available.

Dr Budwig noted that "The formation of tumors usually happens as follows. In those body areas which normally host many growth processes, such as in the skin and membranes, the glandular organs, for example, the liver and pancreas or the glands in the stomach and intestinal tract - it is here that the growth processes are brought to a standstill. Because the dipolarity is missing, due to the lack of electron-rich highly unsaturated fat, the course of growth is disturbed - the surface-active fats are not present; the substance becomes inactive before the maturing and shedding process of the cells ever takes place, which results in the formation of tumors."

In one of her books, Dr Budwig wrote "I often take very sick cancer patients away from hospital where they are said to have only a few days left to live, or perhaps only a few hours. This is mostly accompanied by very good results. The very first thing that these patients and their families tell me is that, in the hospital, it was said that they could no longer urinate or produce bowel movements. They suffered from dry coughing without being able to bring up any mucous. Everything was blocked. It greatly encourages them when suddenly, in all these symptoms, the surface-active fats, with their wealth of electrons, (from the flaxseed oil and cottage cheese mixture), start reactivating the vital functions and the patient immediately begins to feel better".

"I have the answer to cancer, but American doctors won't listen. They come here and observe my methods and are impressed. Then they want to make a special deal so they can take it home and make a lot of money. I won't do it, so I'm blackballed in every country." - Dr Budwig.

As Dr Willner, M.D., Ph.D., author of The Cancer Solution, says, "Numerous, independent clinical studies published in major medical journals worldwide confirm Dr. Budwig's findings…. Over 40 years ago Dr Budwig presented clear and convincing evidence, which has been confirmed by hundreds of other related scientific research papers since, that the essential fatty acids were at the core of the answer to the cancer problem… You will come to your own conclusions as to why this simple effective prevention and therapy has not only been ignored - it has been suppressed!"

In order to make use of this information, we really need to actively manage our nutrition. But we cannot even rely on the nutrient profile of the produce we consume, due to the effects of over farming and food processing.

"Compared to 100 years ago, Omega 3 is down 80%, B vitamins are estimated to be down to about 50% of the daily requirement. Vitamin B6 consumption may be low, as it is removed in grain milling and not replaced. Vitamins B1, B2, B3 and E have also been lost in food processing. Minerals are depleted in a similar way. Fibre is down 75-80%. Antinutrients have increased substantially - saturated fat, 100%; cholesterol, 50%; refined sugar nearly 1000%; salt up to 500%; and funny fat isomers nearly 1,000%." - Dr Rudin.

For more information on Dr Budwig's methodologies and other alternative practitioners visit:

http://www.budwigcenter.com/budwig-protocol.php

and

http://www.CancerUncensored.com/alternative-medicine

Dr Gerson and Gerson Therapy

"Here is a therapy which, despite its considerable drawbacks, can cure some of the most intractable medical conditions known to science. Yet the general public, many of whom will perish from cancer, and those charged with their medical care… have never heard of it!" - Dr Richards and Frank Hourigan.

Gerson therapy is based upon two fundamental aspects - toxicity and deficiency. In order to heal, both of these factors must be dealt with as fast and as effectively as possible.

Deficiency comes from the mass produced, processed and preserved food we eat in our modern diet. Toxicity comes from additives, pesticides, heavy metals and all of the chemicals used in our environment.

"74% of Americans are below daily RDA requirements for magnesium, 55% for iron, 68% calcium, 40% vitamin C, 33% B12, 80% B6, 33% B3, 35% B2, 45% B1, 50% vitamin A. 25-50% of hospital patients suffer from protein calorie malnutrition. Pure malnutrition (cachexia) is responsible for at least 22% and up to 67% of all cancer deaths. Up to 80% of all cancer patients have reduced levels of serum albumin, which is a leading indicator of protein and calorie malnutrition. At least 20% of Americans are clinically malnourished, with 70% being sub-clinically malnourished, and the remaining "chosen few" 10% in good optimal health." — Patrick Quillin, Ph.D.

Simply avoiding anything unnatural and focusing on organic, freshly grown, freshly prepared food at least puts your body in a neutral position to enable healing to take place. When your body starts to break down the poisons it has built up, it is then vital to detoxify, partly with freshly prepared juices and also with coffee enemas.

Dr Gerson also found that part of the healing process cannot be done fast enough without supplementation. Enzymes, and other nutrients need to be supplemented to restore your body to a state prior to the years of neglect it has suffered.

The Gerson Institute uses liver extract, pancreatic enzymes, co-enzyme Q10, and more, to help reverse the damage to the most seriously affected organ systems - which may have been further damaged by mainstream protocols such as chemotherapy.

A British study published in the journal Alternative Therapies in Health and Medicine in 1995, entitled "Five-year survival rates of melanoma patients treated by diet therapy after the manner of Gerson: a retrospective review", showed exceptional results achieved by Gerson therapy.

The five-year absolute survival rates of 153 melanoma patients treated by Gerson therapy were compared with results obtained by conventional medicine (surgery, chemotherapy and radiotherapy).

Of the patients with stages I and II (localised) melanoma, 100% of Gerson's patients survived for five years, compared with 79% who received conventional treatment. Patients with stage IIIa (regionally metastasised) melanoma had an 82% five-year survival rate with Gerson therapy, versus only a 39% five-year survival rate from conventional therapies.

Those patients with combined stages IIIa and IIIb (regionally metastasised) melanoma had a 70% five-year survival rate with Gerson therapy, versus 41% with conventional treatment. Those patients with stage IV (distant metastases), showed a five-year survival rate of 39% with Gerson therapy but only a 6% five-year survival rate with conventional medicine.

With such incredible results, the medical establishment surely showered Dr Gerson with accolades and funding didn't they? No.

"..... no diet has ever been shown to cure cancer." - Barrie Cassileth, Ph.D, American Cancer Society Spokesperson (2007). (It looks like Barrie Cassileth didn't read the study published in Alternative Therapies in Health and Medicine).

After Gerson published his book in 1958, in which he claimed to have cured 50 terminal cancer patients, ("A Cancer Therapy: Results of 50 Cases), the establishment fought back by suspending his medical license. Gerson died in 1959, leaving his daughter Charlotte to continue his work. Charlotte Gerson founded the Gerson Institute in 1977.

According to Maurice Natenberg, in his 1959 book: The Cancer Blackout... "At the time Doctor Gerson testified, he was still on the staff of the Gotham Hospital of New York. Today, he is not on the staff of any hospital. Once he instructed his associates in his method of cancer therapy. Today he finds it impossible to secure medical assistants. Approaching the age of eighty, he now practices alone. For over thirty years he has demonstrated excellent results in treating cancer, his approach is on a highly scientific level, and his credentials are the finest. Yet he has never received a penny to aid in his researches ... Despite the fact that the Gerson therapy is based on authentic physiology, discoveries in biochemistry and nutrition, it has met the usual blackout. The originator is isolated: the medical journals will not publish his work."

S. J. Haught wrote the following in the 1992 book 'Censured for Curing Cancer: The American Experience of Dr. Max Gerson':

"While writing the story of Gerson, I couldn't help feeling it was too shocking to believe. The friends with whom I discussed it became almost angry in their denial that anything of the sort could happen in this day and age. It developed that we were all naïve... there had been dozens of lone scientists... who had been stamped out of existence and driven to spending their last days in solitude and bitterness."

"On two occasions Gerson became violently ill... Lab tests showed... arsenic in his urine. Some of Gerson's best case histories mysteriously disappeared from his files... Gerson was invited on a talk show by host Long John Nebel... Nebel was fired the very next day and the radio network was threatened by the AMA." - Norman Fritz.

The following article by Howard Straus, the grandson of Dr. Max Gerson, (and author of the doctor's biography, Dr. Max Gerson: Healing the Hopeless), says a lot about the politics of the cancer industry and the effectiveness of Gerson therapy:

Censorship, Sports and the Power of One Word

(OMNS May 21, 2012) At the World Snooker Championships, one of the finalists, Peter Ebdon, who had qualified for the Snooker Championship finals an amazing 21 times in a row, was asked to remove a logo from his tee shirt.

Anyone who watches almost any sport at all is certainly familiar with the blizzard of brand name logos for everything from banks to watches, from lubricants to cigarettes, from pain relief medications and golf paraphernalia to the naming of stadia. The commercialization of virtually every sport in this fashion is virtually a "given," no matter how harmful or carcinogenic a product may be, to the extent that it is a multi-billion-dollar a year industry in itself, with star sports figures earning millions of dollars in product endorsements.

But Peter Ebdon raised a firestorm by wearing a logo that said, "Gerson Therapy." Interestingly, few of the photographs of Ebdon in any of the articles clearly showed the logo. Ebdon was moved to wear the logo after his father's death from cancer. But the explosion from the cancer, pharmaceutical and medical industry was prompt. "World Snooker received several messages questioning whether he should be allowed to wear the Gerson Therapy logo," noted the Telegraph newspaper article.

"Obviously, I've upset somebody somewhere, but personally, I think it's too important for people not to know," said Ebdon, in a post-competition press conference. World Snooker officials clearly disagree, justifying their censorship by pointing to a rarely-enforced 1939 law prohibiting the advertising of any cancer therapy, or virtually any public speech about it. This law is never invoked when white-coated oncologists touting toxic chemotherapy or other ineffective but immensely profitable allopathic cancer treatments take to the airwaves.

In a very personal endorsement of Gerson Therapy principles, Ebdon has become a vegan since his father's death.

It is impossible to avoid the parallels to another, similar case. In 2004, when HRH Prince Charles mentioned the word Gerson once in one speech at the Royal College of Gynecology and Obstetrics, the medical and pharmaceutical industry in the UK pilloried him in the tabloid press for months. The Prince had said: "I know of one patient who turned to Gerson Therapy having been told she was suffering from terminal cancer and would not survive another course of chemotherapy. Happily, seven years later, she is alive and well. So it is vital that, rather than dismissing such experiences, we should further investigate the beneficial nature of these treatments." It is not exactly a wild-eyed statement.

Yet attacks on Prince Charles went so far as to imply that the Prince was crazy and lament that royals could no longer be beheaded. The tabloids picked up the story, and ran with it around the world. It was only when they realized that they were exposing the name Gerson to millions of people who would have otherwise never heard of it that they finally went silent.

Now, once again, the name Gerson, put forth publicly by one person, on one occasion, has given the medical/pharmaceutical industry apoplexy, and generated tens of thousands of words of calumny in the controlled press. Many people must be wondering what generated that kind of reaction. This "over-the-top" response is the greatest acknowledgement that the word Gerson clearly generates such fear in the medicine-for-profit industry that its knee-jerk reaction is to spew abuse in all directions.

The pharmaceutical industry is the most profitable business on the face of the planet. Yet it is terrified of one word, whether spoken by a prince or worn by a snooker player. If they have to resort to silencing even the quietest whisper of dissent, they are exposing their lack of confidence in their own competitiveness as providers of methods and products that are supposed to enhance and restore good health.

For more information on Dr Gerson's methodologies and other alternative practitioners visit:

http://www.gerson.org

and

http://www.CancerUncensored.com/alternative-medicine

Dr Andrew Ivy and Krebiozen

"Prior to crossing swords with the FDA in the early 1960s, Dr. Ivy had been widely acknowledged as one of the nation's foremost medical specialists.

As head of the University of Illinois, and with the graduate degrees of Doctor of Philosophy (Ph.D.) and Master of Science (M.S.), he was an American Representative at the Nuremberg trials after World War II in Germany.

The American Medical Association had awarded him bronze, silver, and gold medals in recognition of his outstanding work in the field of medicine. He had written over a thousand articles published in scientific and medical journals. In fact, the FDA itself often had called upon him as an expert to offer medical testimony in court.

But when he began to use an unorthodox approach to cancer therapy, overnight he was branded as a "quack." " - "K-Krebiozen - Key to Cancer?" by Herbert Bailey

According to Herbert Bailey's book, A Matter of Life or Death, The Incredible Story of Krebiozen, and an article in Prevention Magazine, "the story began with the experiments of Dr. Stevan Durovic, a former assistant professor at the University of Belgrade. He came to the United States after several years of experimentation in South America, with a drug which he had discovered and which he believed to be a cure for cancer. Once in the United States he was brought to the attention of Dr. Andrew C. Ivy, a medical researcher of unassailable reputation and gigantic stature in his profession. Dr. Ivy was, at the time, vice president of the University of Illinois, and head of its huge Medical School. His efforts in cancer research had led to his appointment as Executive Director of the National Advisory Cancer Council and he was also a director of the American Cancer Society. An important, a respected, an honored man.

Dr. Ivy became interested in the theory and possibilities shown in Dr. Durovic's substance, Krebiozen, and he decided to test it in the scientific manner his experience had taught him was necessary for an accurate picture of the drug's potential. From the very beginning the results were astounding in their positiveness. Though Krebiozen was used only on persons who had been diagnosed as hopeless and close to death, its remarkable characteristics showed themselves almost at once.

There was a lessening or complete disappearance of pain, and in many cases tumors were dissolved and replaced with healthy tissue. Physicians who were trying it all over the country reported like results. It began to look as though science had finally come up with a weapon against cancer that had a chance to win the fight.

With such a product as a cancer cure, scientific and humanitarian considerations are joined by a third consideration - commercialism. Without a doubt, a cancer cure is worth a lot of money. What victim would not offer all he owns, or all he can borrow for even a chance that he might be cured? Large drug companies have made millions on substances designed to treat diseases far less urgent and wide spread than cancer. This then is why two Chicago businessmen tried to get control of the distribution rights to Krebiozen. When they were refused, they threatened to ruin Krebiozen and everyone connected with it. One of the men who made this threat was the friend of J. J. Moore, then treasurer of the American Medical Association.

The promise shown in the early tests of Krebiozen seemed to be emphasized with each new experiment. The excitement and relief provided by such apparent success left little room for worry over the threat that had been made. How could so proud and secure a venture as a scientifically proven cancer cure be scuttled by the influence of commercial interests?

The answer to that question came with devastating swiftness. In rapid succession Dr. Ivy was suspended from membership in the Chicago Medical Society, removed from the vice presidency of the University of Illinois, and had his resignation accepted by both national cancer societies noted above. But worst of all, his work with Krebiozen was assailed as inaccurate and unscientific. His conclusions were dismissed or so interpreted as to discredit his research methods, methods which had been good enough to earn him a worldwide reputation, methods which till then had been regarded as the ultimate in scientific detachment and objectivity. Suddenly the approach was wrong, the conclusions untrue, the impression was fostered that Dr. Ivy was no longer capable of reliable scientific observation. It was even suggested that Dr. Ivy had become senile and was loyal to Krebiozen only because his mind was failing.

In his book, Fascism in Medicine, Gary Null, Ph.D explains that "over the next three years, Krebiozin was destroyed. But to destroy Krebiozin you first had to destroy Andrew Ivy. How do you destroy the most influential, respected scientist in the United States? You get friends in the media. You get rid of his academic affiliations. You start a whisper campaign. And next thing you know, nobody wants to know the man.

It took about five years, then they brought him up on a trial of fraud. It was, at that point, the longest medical trial in the United States' history. At the end of it, the jury found Ivy and the Durovic brothers innocent. Not only that, but they found the FDA irresponsible. And the jury actually made a statement, which is rare, about the contempt that the FDA had for honesty in what it did at trial."

According to the book, K-Krebiozen - Key to Cancer? by Herbert Bailey, "During the course of Dr. Ivy's trial, a letter was read into the court record written by a doctor from Indianapolis. The doctor stated in his letter that he was treating a patient who had multiple tumors, and that a biopsy of the tissue had shown these tumors to be cancerous. The doctor said that he had obtained Krebiozen from Dr. Ivy's laboratories and had administered it, but that it had done absolutely no good.

When called to the witness stand, however, the doctor's answers were vague and evasive. Under the pressure of cross-examination, he finally broke down and admitted that he never had treated such a patient, never had ordered the biopsy in question, and never had used Krebiozen even once. The whole story had been a lie. Why did he give false testimony? His reply was that one of the FDA agents had written the letter and asked him to sign it. He did so because he wanted to help the agency put an end to quackery.

In September of 1963, the FDA released a report to the effect that Krebiozen was, for all practical purposes, the same as creatine, a common substance that was found in every hamburger. To prove this point, they produced a photographic overlay supposedly showing the spectograms of Krebiozen and creatine superimposed over each other. These were published in Life magazine and other segments of the mass communications media as "unimpeachable proof" that Krebiozen was useless.

When Senator Paul Douglas saw the spectrograms, he was suspicious. So he asked Dr. Scott Anderson, one of the nation's foremost authorities on spectrograms, to make his own study. Using standard techniques of analysis, Dr. Anderson identified twenty-nine differences between the two substances. There were sixteen chemical and color differences. The version released to the press by the FDA had been carefully moved off center until there was a maximum appearance of similarity, but when restored to the true axis, the two were as different as night and day."

Unfortunately, the harmless compound Krebiozen, was, and still is, buried. In fact, the publishers of the book "K-Krebiozen - Key to Cancer" were out of business within a year of publishing it.

Dr. Ivy prepared a monograph in which he reported on 687 patients over a six year period who had been treated with Krebiozen. The work showed observable benefits in 70% of the cases, and directly objective beneficial results in 50% of the cases. He sent an article based on this monograph to one medical journal after another, only to have it returned with apologies and excuses for not being able to publish it.

Dr. Ivy even offered the AMA the opportunity to participate in a double-blind study, with Krebiozen, but using their own selection of Doctors, their own selection of patients, with a public publishing of the results. They refused.

But alas, history is written by the victors, so much of the information you will find on this topic is negative.

Dr Burton's IAT - Immuno-Augmentative Therapy

Dr Lawrence Burton developed a therapy called IAT or immuno-augmentative therapy, which involved the use of serum isolates, cytokines and "immune directive proteins" taken from human patients to stimulate an immune response, and to hopefully restore the body's natural immune defences.

According to the book "Alternatives in Cancer Therapy" by Ross, R.Ph. Pelton and Lee Overholser, "much of Burton's early work was conducted during his fifteen years as a cancer researcher at St. Vincent's Hospital in New York City. In the mid-1960s, Burton and his colleagues made several remarkable presentations at scientific gatherings.

In 1966 an astonished audience at the American Cancer Society's Science Writers' seminar watched as Burton injected blood-derived immunological proteins into mice and caused tumors to shrink in less than one hour.

Several months later, before an audience of oncologists at the New York Academy of Medicine, Dr. Burton and his colleagues reported that the immune factors in the blood that they had discovered were capable of inhibiting cancer. In experiments with leukemic mice, they reported an average survival of 131 days, while untreated mice had an average survival of only 12 days.

At the same meeting, Burton again presented the amazing demonstration of causing tumor masses to visibly shrink within an hour by injecting his "deblocking factor" into tumor-bearing mice. However, instead of being impressed, the audience of oncologists was reportedly skeptical and unconvinced.

Independent mavericks do not usually receive a warm reception from traditional scientists and physicians. Burton's remarkable tumor-shrinking demonstrations before scientific audiences resulted in newspaper headlines that read "15-Minute Cancer Cure." These sensational reports contributed to the American Cancer Society's decision to place immuno-augmentative therapy on the "Unproven Methods" list.

Burton's funding and grant money were withdrawn, and, despite repeated attempts, professional journals refused to publish any more of his papers.

In 1973, with the help of independent funding, Dr. Burton and his associate Dr. Frank Friedman left St. Vincent's and opened the Immunology Research Foundation (IRF) in Great Neck, New York.

Burton and Friedman began treating cancer patients with immuno-augmentative therapy at the clinic. They also applied for and obtained U.S. patents on the four proteins that they had isolated from human blood. These substances were called deblocking protein (DP), tumor antibody 1 (TA1), tumor antibody 2 (TA2), and tumor complement (TC). Burton claimed that when these substances are used in the right combination, they can restore the normal immune function in cancer patients.

During this period Burton and Friedman had also applied to the FDA for an Investigational New Drug (IND) permit. When it became obvious that they could not satisfy the FDA's seemingly endless requests for more information and additional studies, Burton and Friedman closed their New York research facility.

In 1977 Dr. Burton branched out on his own and moved to the city of Freeport, on Grand Bahama Island, where he opened the Immunology Research Centre (IRC). A steady stream of cancer patients began traveling to the Bahamas, and for several years things went well for Burton.

Then, in July 1985, Burton was hit with another serious challenge. With urging from the National Cancer Institute and several other U.S. health agencies, the Bahamian government forced Burton to close his clinic because of reported AIDS and hepatitis B viral contamination of his blood-derived products.

Two authors who summarized the events leading to the closing of Burton's clinic questioned the validity of the charges. Dr. Harold Jaffe, then director of the AIDS program at the Centers for Disease Control, pointed out that the wrong test was used to evaluate Burton's material. The ELISA test, which was used in the investigation, produces large numbers of false positive results. Another, more accurate test, which was readily available, was not used.

In February 1986, an article appeared in the AMA journal stating that all the gamma-globulin samples in the U.S. had been contaminated with the AIDS antibody. At the same time, AIDS test kits revealed that thousands of blood samples from blood centers around the United States tested positive for the AIDS virus. None of these centers were closed.

One has to wonder why several U.S. agencies singled out Burton's clinic for closing for a health problem that was affecting every major medical institution and blood bank throughout the United States.

Robert Houston, an authority on alternative cancer therapies, states that "the overkill regarding Burton's clinic was clearly an attempt to play up any excuse to have it closed." In March 1986, after evaluating all the evidence that had surfaced, the Bahamian Ministry of Health reversed its decision and allowed Burton to reopen his clinic.

The closing of Burton's clinic enraged his patients and their families. Many of these people joined to form the Immuno-Augmentative Therapy Patient Association (IATPA) and began to lobby members of the U.S. Congress for help. The controversy over IAT was primarily responsible for persuading Congress to order the OTA study of alternative cancer therapies.

Dr. Burton's clinic continues to operate successfully in the Bahamas. He does not claim that his immuno-augmentative therapy is a cure for cancer. Instead, he believes that IAT is an immune-system-enhancing therapy that is often successful in controlling cancer. Although Burton's results have not been independently verified, the IAT patient brochure claims that from 50 to 60 percent of the patients experience a reduction in tumor size, and that many achieve long-term remission."

As part of his research into Dr. Burton's work, Gary Null Ph.D. noted, "We went through the records and we found over five hundred of his patients who were alive and well five years after their treatment, with no cancer. And Dr. Burton didn't selectively give us these. These were "take what you want. Here are the patients I treated." So there was statistical improvement - more so than any cancer institution in the United States could show."

"The survival rate of Dr Burton's patients approximately doubled the maximum survival rate of conventionally treated patients.

Had these findings pertained to a chemotherapy drug instead of IAT, massive amounts of funding would have been allocated to investigate the drug. Once again, the politics of cancer barred a potentially valuable treatment from reaching the public." - J. Diamond, M.D.

Dr Burton died in 1993, but his clinic is still operated by his trusted colleagues:

http://immunemedicine.com

Dr. Royal R. Rife - every disease has a frequency

Dr. Royal R. Rife discovered that every disease has a frequency which can be measured. He also discovered that different foods and essential oils carry different frequencies and could therefore be used to influence the frequencies found in our body.

The healthy human body carries a frequency of 62 to 68 MHz, whereas cancer only has a frequency of 42 MHz or less.

"In every culture and in every medical tradition before ours, healing was accomplished by moving energy." - Albert Szent-Gyorgyi, Nobel Laureate in Medicine (1937).

What Rife proved is that every health disorder has a frequency, which in turn responds, or resonates, to a specific and optimal frequency for its dissolving / healing in the body.

With this discovery, Dr Rife developed a series of machines which could emit these specific frequencies as part of a treatment.

According to www.Rife.org, "Another doctor and scientist, whose research has been buried for some time but has managed to resurface due to the work of avid supporters, is Dr Royal Raymond Rife M.D, who developed a frequency generator in the late 1920's. In brief, Rife successfully treated 1,000 patients diagnosed with incurable cancer in the 1930's. He was honoured with 14 awards and an honorary doctorate.

After the unsuccessful attempt by pharmaceutical companies to buy out his research and equipment, his office was ransacked, his research paperwork was stolen and the machine that healed all those 1,000 "incurable" cancer patients was destroyed.

In 1934, before this destruction occurred, the University of Southern California appointed a Special Medical Research Committee to bring terminal cancer patients from Pasadena County Hospital to Rife's San Diego Laboratory and clinic for treatment. The team included doctors and pathologists assigned to examine the patients - if still alive - in 90 days. After the 90 days of treatment, the Committee concluded that 86.5% of the patients had been completely cured. The treatment was then adjusted and the remaining 13.5% of the patients also responded within the next four weeks. The total recovery rate using Rife's technology was 100%."

According to Barry Lynes, author of The Cancer Cure That Worked!, "Milbank Johnson, M.D conducted... [a] study of the Rife Frequency Generator as a potential cancer treatment. Dr Johnson coordinated the study in conjunction with the Medical Research Committee of the University of Southern California. He treated 16 patients with various types of advanced cancers, all of whom had been declared "terminal" or "incurable". After 3 months of the Rife treatment, 14 of these "hopeless" cases were declared clinically cured and in good health by a staff of 5 M.D.'s and by Alvin G Ford, M.D. group pathologist.

Dr Johnson died in 1944. The suspicion exists that he was silenced... However two federal inspectors did examine his hospital record in the late 1950's. They concluded it was likely that he was poisoned.

A number of subsequent clinics in the years 1935-1938 accomplished similar cures... the AMA virtually stopped the Rife treatment in 1939, first by threatening the physicians using Rife's instrument, then by forcing Rife into court... During the period 1935 to early 1939, the leading laboratory for electronic or energy medicine in the USA, in New Jersey, was independently verifying Rife's discoveries... this laboratory was 'mysteriously' burned to the ground.... Rife's treatment was ruthlessly suppressed by the AMA's Morris Fishbein."

Even now, Rife-type technology is being targeted by the FDA in order to stamp it out. According to Cindy Charlebois, "My good friend Jim Folsom (Global Wellness Rife-type device distributor), is in jail awaiting sentencing. There was a federal jury trial and he was convicted of 26 felony counts relating to his sale of "unapproved" medical devices.

This is so WRONG!

Jim is a very, very good man. He has hundreds (if not thousands) of testimonials where his devices improved symptoms, and in many cases seemed to actually clear up many health problems. He helped so many people. In my case, my father-in-law who had prostate cancer improved his PSA score from 70 down to 0.5 (YES, that's zero point five) in 2.5 months using the Global Wellness device and taking B17. My (19-year-old) daughter had bullous impetigo which she cleared without prescription drugs using the Global Wellness device and a terminator zapper. Go to the www.rifeforum.com and look for the "CindyCharlebois" (my user name on that forum) posts for details.

According to the Official US Attorney's News Release, he was found guilty of 26 felony charges possibly resulting in a maximum sentencing time of 140 years, and up to a $500,000 fine."

For more information, on Dr Rife and his work, visit:

http://www.rife.org/

and

http://www.CancerUncensored.com/alternative-medicine

Dr. William Koch and Glyoxylide

"During his lifetime, Dr. William F. Koch presented to the world medical community a new method for the treatment of cancer and its allied diseases, based upon his research and studies of the body's natural immune system." - The Koch Family.

Dr Koch discovered a distinction between cancer patients and healthy individuals. Cancer patients had high levels of a substance called guanidine in their tissues. Dr Koch could not detect guanidine in any healthy tissue, so he theorised that it must be being converted from a hormone called methyl-cyanamide and that the body normally detoxifies and eliminates this harmful substance, if it creates it at all.

He realised that if he could prevent this conversion process, by using a proprietary substance that binds cyanamide, then he could have an impact upon cancer.

According to Dr Koch, "This substance when purified, taken up in water and immediately injected subcutaneously into a cancer patient, causes practically no local reaction; but instead, after about 24 hours, a very decided focal reaction takes place. Wherever the cancer tissue may be, its cells are killed, their ionic concentration increases, the osmotic pressure increases, they take up water, swell and disintegrate. The swelling causes pain and the absorbed, disintegrated products are oxidized causing fever.

Those two things, focal pain and fever, constitute a reaction which lasts all the way from 6 to 48 hours, depending upon the amount of cancer tissue killed, and of course this depends upon the quantity of substance injected. Such a reaction occurs only in cancer cases and only in the presence of cancer tissue. After the cancer tissue has disappeared, no more reaction can be elicited, no matter how large an injection is given, an important diagnostic aid.

The specificity of the substance for cancer is evidenced by the fact that while giving these injections in rapid succession (that is daily or every two days for a period of five weeks), a blood count will rise from 2,850,000 to 4,600,000 red cells and the haemeglobin from 37% to 82%. Thus the delicate red cells are not injured. At the same time a mass of cancer tissue, up to the size of a large cabbage, will entirely disappear, and all the signs and symptoms of the particular cancer will disappear with it, function return, and the patient become clinically cured.

Stomach, liver and rectal cancers clear up the quickest. Uterus cancer responds slightly more slowly. Squamous cell carcinoma responds about one-half as fast as stomach cancer. No cases of cancer that have previously received X-ray or Radium treatment respond to this treatment at all since these agencies have altered the chemistry of the cancer cell. I therefore, cannot make any statements regarding breast cancer, since those breast cases that I have treated have all been previously rayed.

Before presenting a few brief case descriptions, I wish to express my gratitude and appreciation to Dr. Carstens, Dr. Judd, Dr. Paterson, Dr. Irvine, Dr. Palmerlee, Dr. Palmer, Dr. Blain, Dr. Watkins, Dr. Hewitt, Dr. Friedlander, Dr. Hackett, Dr. John Burleson, Dr. Ash, Dr. Van Baalen, Dr. Hurst, for the excellent cases they have offered and for their kind co-operation in the treatments of their cases. I think that interviewing them would prove more interesting and instructive than any mass of details that I could here append.

It appears from these brief case histories, that each injection does its work and that the growth does not become immune to the treatment, that destruction of the cancer removes all its noxious activities as eroding blood vessels, nerves, etc., and that the toxic products are no longer generated, so that the cachecia disappears and a return to the normal strength, body weight and blood count ensue."

"I had a woman patient last August, with a cancerous growth as large as a watermelon. She was too weak to walk and wanted to live only until her son returned from France. I did not expect her to live a week. Today she is as well as any of us. It is the same with all stomach cases I have treated; they are either entirely well or getting well as quickly as treatment proceeds. And the same is true of rectum or uterus cancer that have not been treated with X-ray or radium."

- William F. Koch, Ph.D., M.D., Professor of Physiology, Detroit College of Medicine and Surgery; Research Pathologist to the Woman's Hospital; Director of Laboratory to the Jefferson Clinic.

Over time, Dr Koch studied over two dozen different related substances, trying to find the most effective compounds.

According to Dr. Alexander W. Blain, surgeon and head of Jefferson clinic, "Dr. Koch is one of the most brilliant physiological chemists in the country. It is too early to say he has a cancer cure, and it should not be regarded as a 'cure-all' but as an adjunct to the treatment of cancer. No cure can be established until five years have shown there is no recurrence of the disease. But what he has done is this: He has made people well who were so far gone with cancer that they had only a few weeks to live.

Several patients he treated for me are working hard and enjoying life a year after they 'should have been dead.' Even if Dr. Koch gets no further with his work than he is now – and he is experimenting now with his fifteenth mixture, I believe – even if he has not discovered an absolute cure for cancer, he has added years to the lives of cancer victims. There are nearly 300,000 victims of cancer in the country and if they could all have a few years of usefulness added to their lives the saving to the country would be enormous. What he has already done is a boon to humanity and a great step forward in physiological chemistry."

Dr. Walter L. Hackett, gynecologist and obstetrician, was amongst many other medical professionals who also endorsed Dr Kochs's work, saying "There is no question of Dr. Koch's sincerity and ability. It will take five years to determine whether or not he has a real cure for cancer, but I have enough confidence in his treatment to let him inject his serum into any cancer patient of mine. I had, as a patient, an old woman who was very far-gone. At Koch's suggestion I operated on her and took out such cancerous growths as were apparent. Later, the cancer grew again. Dr. Koch gave her four injections and she is now apparently entirely well. I have seen some excellent work done with radium, but never anything so remarkable as this. Dr. Koch should be given every opportunity to prove the value of his treatment."

Despite Dr Koch's promising work and the co-operation of numerous oncologists, who had seen the results of his work first-hand, Dr Koch was unable to secure funding or facilities to further his research.

But he did conclude that there was one specific enzyme reaction in cells which could be corrupted to trigger a cascade of unnecessary cell replication. He believed that his most effective compound, which he called glyoxylide, with its high electron activity, could potentially donate electrons to reverse this problem.

Strangely enough, this meant that despite being decades apart and working from totally different approaches, Dr Rife, Dr Budwig and Dr Koch all had arrived at the conclusion that cancer could be an issue of the electrical charge or action of electrons on cells.

Unfortunately, in keeping with many other pioneers of cancer research, Dr Koch was eventually sued by the FDA, but was acquitted after more than 600 doctors testified in his favour. He died of poisoning in 1967.

In a letter from Willard H. Dow, President of Dow Chemical Company, dated June 21, 1946, to Mr. Laurence B. Thatcher, Dr. Dow wrote the following about Dr Koch:

"His recent trial in connection with the Pure Food and Drug Administration has brought him the support of some of our technical people on the basis of submitting technical information that is available here and has been proved up and which the government had attempted to misrepresent. Our intention all the way through has been to try to get at the truth of this whole matter, and whether it is Dr. Koch or somebody else, we would take the same attitude to try to prevent an innocent man from being crucified.

We cannot understand what the Food and Drug Administration is driving at for the reason that all our information to date would indicate Dr. Koch has been exonerated from illegal practices as far as the Administration is concerned, and as for the mislabeling of packages, like everyone else it is merely a matter of interpretation rather than willful violation of the law. Before the present trial came up, Dr. Koch had appeared before the Washington representatives of this department and thought the whole matter was straightened out to their satisfaction, but apparently not so.

It is strange, because the same procedure is run into time and time again by industry when it is necessary to get a label properly approved before it goes to the public, but in his case it does not seem to be possible without a trial. He has had no trouble in proving his points, but the government has spent a tremendous amount of moncy to try to prove he is wrong. It almost sounds as if a certain group is attempting to persecute him unjustly."

"In 1926...The AMA attempted to send a doctor using Koch shots to prison... in Massachusetts... Justice Pierce berated the District Attorney, calling the opposition to Koch 'a moral crime of the very worst kind'." "One doctor, J.W. Kannel, saved a young girl. She had hopeless cancer of the spleen... One shot of Glyoxylide, and she became well (in 1943; still alive in 1983)... For this,

Kannel was barred from all hospitals in Fort Wayne... The FDA had Glyoxylide inventor, Dr. William Frederick Koch arrested and thrown into an incredibly filthy jail cell in Florida in 1942." - Wayne Martin BS, Purdue Univ. (Author, Medical Heroes and Heretics); We Can Do Without Heart Attacks. c. 1983.

"Dr. Koch himself was the target of at least 13 unsuccessful attempts on his life' - Riley H. Crabb." - M. Layne, The Koch Remedy for Cancer, Borderland Sciences Research Foundation.

Unfortunately, the secret of Dr Koch's reagents died with him, and all that remains are the attempts to discredit him.

Dr Koch had publicly stated, "I do not want to make the formula public just yet, because I fear it might be commercialized. The compound is difficult to make and it deteriorates rapidly. If I published it and quacks or unscientific men started mixing it and treating cancer with it, the results would be disastrous, not only possibly to the patients, but to the ultimate success of the treatment. Improperly mixed or administered, the compound would fail to do its work. It would be discredited by the medical profession and it would take years to establish its value. When I have proved to the satisfaction of the medical world that it does its work, it will be time enough to make the formula public."

And so a potential weapon against cancer was lost.

"After failing in its attempt to gain sole control over his research, Organized Medicine launched a fifty-year, unlimited assault aimed at discrediting Dr. Koch's reputation, medical practice and research, along with those of any physician who dared to validate his Theories or use his Reagents. Organized Medicine developed an extensive propaganda campaign, disseminated false information on Reagent chemistry and publicly dismissed the Koch Theories, which emphasized the relationship between environmental toxins, dietary deficiencies and a depleted oxidation mechanism, as primary initiators of the disease process.

Because Dr. Koch endured such extensive persecution in regard to his science, he determined that the medical/pharmacological industry would forever remain unwilling to independently monitor, document or validate any of his ongoing laboratory research or medical case histories; therefore since his death, December 9, 1967, there have been no authentic Koch Reagents reproduced." - The Koch Family, http://www.williamfkoch.com

Please see:

http://www.williamfkoch.com

or

http://www.CancerUncensored.com/alternative-medicine

Ozone therapy and Oxygen Therapy

Ozone therapy is used at many cancer centres in Germany. Not only does ozone kill cancer cells, but it kills viruses and bacteria too.

The therapy involves a small measure of your blood being taken, infused with ozone, then fed back into a vein via a drip. This has the effect of hyper oxygenating the blood, which is highly detrimental to cancer cells and viruses.

It is not an isolated treatment - it is used as part of a suite of complementary therapies which create an increasingly harsh environment for cancer cells to live in.

"The FDA won't spend a dime on ozone research, but they spent over $1 million intimidating, harassing, and persecuting me alone." - Dr Jonathan Wright

According to www.whale.to, "Dr. F.M. Eugene Blass, developer of "Homozon™" (the original oxygen therapy product) was murdered outside his house, the same year and month as Dr Koch. Dr Basil Earle Wainright, a Physicist and inventor of polyatomic apheuresis oxygen therapy was imprisoned for 4 years. He claims he survived six assassination attempts whilst in prison.

Dr George A. Freibott, IV, the President of the American Naturopathic Association, a consultant for the International Association for Oxygen Therapy, a US Government approved and internationally accepted expert witness on oxygen / oxidation therapies, survived numerous assassination attempts and several anonymous phone calls threatening his life."

Dietary and intravenous vitamin C or ascorbic acid.

Vitamin C is found in numerous fruits and vegetables and is vital for our survival. The richest sources include blackcurrants, guava, red peppers, oranges and other citrus fruit, papaya, strawberries, tomatoes, broccoli, potatoes and more.

On top of being an excellent antioxidant, vitamin C is used in the production of collagen (required for skin, bone, muscle, tendons, ligaments and blood vessels). It is also required in the production of some of your neurotransmitters and the synthesis of carnitine, which helps convert fat into energy in your cells. Vitamin C is also needed to convert cholesterol into bile acid.

As with many other vitamins and minerals, there is a recommended daily allowance of vitamin C.

Current dietary recommended daily allowances, (RDAs), for vitamins and minerals, relate to the bare minimum quantities necessary to prevent deficiency diseases, such as scurvy.

The RDAs are not set at what is required for optimum health. That is a big difference.

Neil Riordan at the Riordan Clinic, Arizona noted that 46 per cent of breast cancer sufferers are vitamin C deficient, some even to the point of scurvy (British Journal of Cancer Vol 84, II).

It is theorised that during the course of our evolution, we lost one of the 4 enzymes necessary to manufacture vitamin C within our own bodies, so we must consume it as part of our diet. Animals, (except for guinea pigs), are able to make their own.

Interestingly, if you look at the amount of vitamin C per kg of body weight across all animals, it is very similar, from a mouse to an elephant. It equates to what would be around a 1500mg daily dose for an adult human.

Yet the UK RDA for vitamin C in people is only set at 60mg, or 1/25th of the level that every other mammal on this planet has in their bodies. The US RDA is set at 75mg for men and 90mg for women.

More shockingly, these levels were determined by the National Institute of Health after just 2 studies involving only 7 and 15 participants respectively!

I find it disgusting that they can dictate the safe daily consumption of a vital nutrient for 300 million people, (and all of their future offspring), based upon data from just 22 people!

A case in point is that 35% of our population require more vitamin C than usual due to the depleting effects of smoking, the contraceptive pill, pregnancy, diabetes and using aspirin or numerous other drugs.

Is it any wonder that our immune systems fail and that our arteries become decreasingly elastic from reducing levels of collagen and elastin, because you need vitamin C in order to make them.

You really cannot take it for granted that mainstream science has all the answers. The bogus RDAs issued by the NIH have probably cost millions of lives.

An epidemiological study published in the American Journal of Clinical Nutrition, by the NIH in the year 2000, showed that adults whose blood plasma concentrations exceeded the 73.8 micromole level [equivalent to a 500-1000mg daily dose] experienced a 57 percent reduced risk of dying from any cause and a 62 percent reduced relative risk of dying of cancer when compared to adults who consumed low amounts of vitamin C (28 micromole) [equivalent to the RDA].

Have they changed the RDA for vitamin C in light of this research? No.

Another study, published in the journal Epidemiology in 1998, demonstrated that for every 500 microgram increase in blood serum level of vitamin C, an 11 percent reduction in coronary heart disease and stroke prevalence could be anticipated.

A firm advocate of a higher vitamin C RDA, Dr. Hickey, estimates that 500mg of vitamin C, taken orally in 5 divided doses every three waking hours daily, (2500mg total per day), could reduce the cardiovascular mortality risk by 55 percent compared with people consuming low doses of vitamin C.

According to the Journal of the American College of Nutrition, 1995, eight different double-blind, placebo-controlled studies and six non-placebo controlled clinical trials have confirmed the safety of vitamin C, where up to 10,000mg of vitamin C was consumed daily for up to 3 years.

Just take a look at the research on the impact of 2000 to 2500mg daily vitamin C:

- The reduction of, and delay of, forming cataracts (J Clinical Epidemiology 52: 1207-11, 1999; Am J Clin Nutrition 66: 911-16, 1997)

- Reduction in the symptoms of arthritis (Arthritis Rheumatism 39: 648-56, 1996)
- People getting colds less often and for a shorter duration (Advances Therapy 19: 151-59, 2002)
- Smokers living longer, with less symptoms (J Am College Nutrition 22: 372-78, 2003)
- Rates of gall bladder disease dropping by 25% (J Clinical Epidemiology 51: 257-65, 1998)
- 2.68 times less calcification of arteries (American Journal of Epidemiology, 2004)
- The risk of angina in adults who consume high levels of alcohol cut by half (Ann Epidemiology. 9: 358-65, 1999)
- A 750mg daily dose of vitamin C could increase male life-span by 6 years (Epidemiology 3: 194-202, 1992)

But these levels are very difficult to achieve with diet alone. So in order to have the raw building blocks necessary for health, and to act as an antioxidant, vitamin C supplementation should be considered a necessity.

In the past, high doses of vitamin C have been shown in studies to eliminate the risk of cot death, reverse heart disease, destroy certain viruses, and now it has been strongly linked with killing cancer cells, especially if given intravenously.

But the integration of Vitamin C into cancer treatment has not been at all smooth, despite the compelling evidence. Perhaps this is because it is very cheap to produce, not patentable and hard to monetise. So just like many other "alternative" medicines, the cancer establishment has resisted it ferociously.

According to CANCERactive, a UK holistic cancer charity, "In 1974, Cameron and Campbell took 50 terminal cancer patients and gave them 10 grams intravenously of sodium ascorbate (a form of vitamin C). All had been given less than three months to live. Half survived 361 days on average with five people surviving an average of 610 days.

They requested that the National Cancer Institute conduct proper clinical trials - a double blind study. For some reason this was denied.

So Linus Pauling and Cameron repeated the experiment with 100 terminal cancer patients, comparing them with control groups of 1000 people in all. Whilst all the 1000 control group died, 18 of the group receiving vitamin C survived, and five of these appeared to overcome the disease.

In 1978, Pauling and Cameron repeated this in a second study, this time taking nine control groups each with similar cancers to the test group. As in the previous tests, the patients taking intravenous vitamin C had renewed vigour and energy and their quality of life improved. Whilst all of the control group died, the vitamin C group lived 300 days on average and five patients survived for 16 months."

As a result of these studies, Ewan Cameron and the two-time Nobel Prize winner, Linus Pauling, concluded that intravenous vitamin C could significantly increase the cancer patient's life-span.

Three subsequent studies, which supposedly replicated their work did not get the same results and were often used to discredit their findings.

Further investigation revealed that the studies used oral doses of vitamin C and not intravenous doses. This is a blatant error, given that for every 1g of vitamin C taken orally, only 7% of it typically makes it into your bloodstream.

A second issue was that Pauling had noted that megadoses of vitamin C did not have anywhere near the same impact upon patients who had previously had chemotherapy. Therefore, when the Mayo clinic replicated the study with 60 patients, where 52 had received chemotherapy, it was no wonder that they did not get the same impressive results.

Unfortunately, such contradictory studies detracted from the message that vitamin C could be highly beneficial in the treatment of cancer.

Given the inability of the body to absorb dietary vitamin C efficiently, Linus Pauling later advocated oral consumption of vitamin C in doses as high as 3 to 6g per day for adults. This is the same as 3000 to 6000mg.

Most people can easily tolerate upwards of 4000mg spread over the day without suffering loose stools from excessive vitamin C intake.

Whilst I would not suggest a dose this high, it is important to realise that vitamin C in your bloodstream only has a half life of around 30 minutes. This means that after 30 minutes, the level of vitamin C in your bloodstream drops in half. In order to counteract this, dividing your vitamin C intake throughout the day is a wise precaution, along with using timed release vitamin tablets.

In addition, co-factors like bioflavinoids increase the effectiveness of vitamin C, so getting your vitamin C from fruit and vegetables, or a supplement which also includes them is wise.

The 1000mg vitamin C tablets I take also contain citrus bioflavinoids and are designed to release over the course of 6 hours. Alternatively, you could eat an orange when you take your tablets.

A gentle word of warning though. If you do consider taking higher doses of vitamin C, you should also increase your magnesium intake to decrease the small possibility of kidney stones. This possibility has largely been debunked, but the magnesium may act as a safeguard just in case.

For more information on this, please visit:

http://www.CancerUncensored.com/recommended-products

Subsequent studies have helped to reinforce the dramatic cancer prevention qualities of vitamin C. Higher levels of blood vitamin C reduce cancer risk for breast, cervix, colon, rectum, mouth, lung, prostate, stomach and oesophagus.

But there have been fears that the FDA are taking steps to ban the intravenous use of vitamin C, even though it is an acknowledged burn treatment in many countries, including the US.

Fortunately, the Center for New Medicine in Irvine, California, has FDA approval to treat cancer patients with vitamin C in trials, so hopefully the resulting published data will stimulate the wider use of this treatment.

At the center, they are using intravenous high dose vitamin C, then enhancing the effect by putting people in a hyperbaric chamber. This means that when the tumour absorbs the vitamin C and produces hydrogen peroxide, the pressure prevents it from actually processing the hydrogen peroxide, which poisons the mechanisms within the cancer cells, triggering programmed cell death. This means that the vitamin C is able to have an anti-cancer effect whilst simultaneously having an immune system stimulating effect.

"Amazingly, vitamin C has actually already been documented in the medical literature to have regularly and consistently cured both acute polio and acute hepatitis, two viral diseases still considered by modern medicine to be incurable." - Thomas E. Levy, M.D., JD

Hyperthermia

It has been documented in numerous studies, that not only is cancer vulnerable to an alkaline pH and high levels of oxygen, but cancer cells are also more vulnerable to heat than healthy cells.

If you heat up tissue enough to kill the cancer cells, but not enough to damage the healthy tissue, you have a targeted therapy.

The reason heat kills cancer cells and not healthy cells is that cancer cells derive their energy from a fermentation process which occurs in cells at lower levels of oxygen. When heat is applied to a cancer cell, it speeds up the rate at which it ferments to produce energy. This generates acidic waste products at a rate which is too fast for the cell to remove them, so it is killed by its own metabolic products. This is called acidosis.

The heat also stimulates tumour cells to release specific proteins onto their outer membranes, which enable our immune system to recognise them as cancer cells - thereby triggering our natural immune response against them.

Local hyperthermia can heat up a localised tumour, but if the cancer has spread, (or is harder to isolate), whole-body hyperthermia can create an artificial fever to cause a generalised response.

Local hyperthermia, brought about by a radio emitter fed into a catheter for 3 hours, has proven to be very effective at treating prostate cancer at centres in Germany, (such as the Klinik St. Georg in Bad Aibling, South Germany), with literally thousands of patients symptom-free years later.

In some centres, they can also combine this with added intravenous vitamin C, selenium, and zinc to help stimulate a greater immune response.

Proteolytic enzymes

An excess of undigested proteins from cooked animal products collects in our digestive tract. If it is allowed to remain there, it ferments and releases toxins into our bloodstream.

If we ate raw food, which is rich in enzymes, this would be less likely to occur. However, in order to beat the buildup we have already exposed ourselves to, we need to supplement our diet with proteolytic digestive enzymes .

Visit:

http://www.CancerUncensored.com/recommended-products

Pancreatic enzymes

Pancreatic enzyme therapy was first used by John Beard in 1902, where he injected pancreatic extracts directly into tumours.

High doses of pancreatic enzymes can break down and digest the protein layer that surrounds a tumour and masks it from our immune system.

As individual cancer cells, our immune system can detect and destoy them, but once a tumour is formed, it becomes much harder for the immune system to detect the cancer in the first place.

"Professor Friedrich Douwes reported over a dozen (pancreas cancer) cures with his biologic therapy, and enzymologist Karl Ransberger had reported on 38 cases of total remission (collected by no less an official than the Austrian minister of health) using his world renowned Wobe-Mugos enzyme." - Dr Atkins.

Alkaline Water

Our bodies are made up of almost 70% water. Healthy blood pH is around 7.35 to 7.45, which is slightly alkaline. However, many of the foods we eat and many of the environmental factors we are exposed to are acidic. Therefore, we need alkaline substances in our diet to help us balance the pH of our bodies.

In the absence of balance, the body draws calcium from our teeth and bones to neutralise the acid in our blood. This is one of the reasons why sugar rots your teeth. It also rots your bones!

Even if your fizzy drinks were put straight into your stomach via a tube, you would still get tooth decay, because in order to neutralise the carbonic acid, your body would draw the calcium from your teeth.

We simply do not have enough calcium reserves to cope with it all, which is why many elderly suffer from osteoporosis.

Prescription drugs, smoking, meat, dairy, some nuts, sugar and wheat all increase the acidity of your body. A significant problem with this is that cancer thrives in an acidic environment.

So not only should we avoid carbonated drinks, we should actively try to repair the pH balance by drinking alkaline water.

You can buy machines that you can hook up to your kitchen tap so that it...

1. filters the water, (to remove heavy metals, bacteria, pesticides and various other toxins),
2. adds minerals to it,
3. processes it to make it a pH of 8 or greater, adding hydrogen (which easily donates its electrons), and
4. reduces the molecule cluster size, (making it more easily absorbable for better hydration).

We know that having a negative charge, (from electrons), is important to the membranes of our cells, because they use the variation in charge, (from the positively charged nucleus to the negatively charged exterior of the cell), to move waste out of the cell and to bring nutrition in.

Therefore, not only do we make our body more hostile to cancer by consuming more alkaline substances, but the extra electrons available from alkaline water help to restore the charge to our cell membranes. Cancer cells have a negative charge on their cell membranes that is three times lower than healthy cells.

Consuming alkaline water also helps to destroy free radicals in your bloodstream before they have chanced to damage your cells. This makes alkaline water somewhat of an antioxidant.

Interestingly, you can see some videos of the before and after effects of alkaline water on YouTube. In particular videos of the insides of people's colons after using this water. It is amazing what water can do for your health. They even use alkaline water to kill E. coli and salmonella in chicken processing plants.

There are several places in the world that people flock to for miraculous healing water, such as the springs of Lourdes in France, the caves of Nordenau in Germany, the wells of Tlacote in Mexico and more.

Interestingly, scientific research conducted by Dr Shirahata of Kyushu University in Japan, shows that these "miraculous" sources of water contain as much as 200 to 300 times more hydrogen than normal tap water.

I have ordered a KeoSan Alkaline Hydrogen Water Filtration System because it infuses tap water with abundant hydrogen.

Further research has also been conducted into the energetic levels of water. It appears that water has some form of energetic memory. Still and dead water has larger clusters of molecules and low energy. But if the water is vortexed, or falls down a waterfall, it ends up with smaller clusters of molecules and greater levels of energy in it.

Interestingly, this makes it a better solvent, so it can remove waste better or transport nutrients more effectively. If you shake a drink that has settled, it mixes up again. This is the same principle.

Not only does the KeoSan machine filter out unwanted impurities, re-mineralise and alkalinise the water, but it also vortexes it to help it to form hexagonal clusters of energised water that are better absorbed.

There are other brands out there, but for less than £200 or $300, this brand seemed excellent value for money, considering its unique features.

Learn more at:

http://www.CancerUncensored.com/recommended-products

Alkaline Forming Foods

If you do not have an alkaline water machine, you can manipulate the pH of your body with what you eat and drink. Different foods, when they are digested, will have the tendency to shift your body towards being more acidic (bad), or more alkaline (good).

Strangely enough, it is not whether the food itself is alkaline or acidic, it is what it does to you AFTER it has been digested. For example, lemons are acidic, and yet they have a very alkalising effect on the human body after digestion.

The following list is not exhaustive, but it helps to show which foods make your body more acidic and which foods make you more alkaline.

Experts recommend a diet of 30% acid forming foods and 70% alkaline forming foods to maintain health, or a diet of 20% acidic and 80% alkaline foods if you are trying to recover your health.

Fruit:

Alkaline forming - apples, apricots, avocado, bananas, berries, cherries, citrus fruit (lemons, limes, oranges, grapefruit), coconuts, dried fruit (dates, figs, prunes, raisins) fresh figs, grapes, kiwifruit, mangoes, melons (cantaloupe, honey dew, watermelon), nectarines, olives*, papayas, peaches, pears, persimmons, plums, tomatoes.

Acid forming - canned fruit, cranberries, glazed fruit, pomegranates, rhubarb, strawberries*.

Vegetables:

All vegetables are alkaline forming - alfalfa, barley grass, broccoli, cabbage, carrots, cauliflower, celery, cucumber, garlic, green beans, kale, lettuce, mushrooms, onions, peas, peppers, pumpkin, radishes, sea vegetables, spinach, sprouts, squash, sweet potatoes, wheatgrass, wild greens.

Nuts:

Alkaline forming - almonds, almond milk, Brazil nuts, chestnuts.

Acid forming - cashews, filberts, macadamias, peanuts, peanut butter, pecans, roasted nuts, tahini, walnuts.

Seeds:

Alkaline forming - all sprouted seeds, cumin seeds, fennel seeds.

Acid forming - chia, flax*, pumpkin*, sesame*, sunflower*.

Beans and peas:

Alkaline forming - all sprouted beans, limas, soybeans, soymilk*, mung beans, white beans.

Acid forming - aduki, kidney, lentils, Navy.

Grains:

Alkaline forming - all sprouted grains, amaranth, buckwheat, corn, millet, quinoa*, rice milk*.

Acid forming - barley, breads, brown rice, oats, processed grain, rye, wheat.

Seasonings, Condiments and Dressings:

Alkaline forming - chilli pepper, cinnamon, curry, ginger, herbs (all), miso, mustard, sea salt, table salt (sodium chloride), Tamari.

Acid forming - jams, ketchup, mayonnaise, mustard, soy sauce, vinegar.

Meat and dairy:

Alkaline forming - goats milk, non-fat organic milk.

Acid forming - all animal meats, butter, cheese, eggs, fish, ice cream, milk, poultry, yoghurt.

Sugars:

Alkaline forming - honey, Stevia.

Acid forming - alcohol of any kind, artificial sweeteners, brown sugar, cane sugar, carob, malt sugar, maple syrup*, milk sugar, white sugar.

Oils:

Alkaline forming - olive oil*, soy oil*, flaxseed oil*.

Acid forming - avocado oil, butter, canola oil, corn oil, cream, hemp seed oil, nut oils, safflower oil, Sesame seed oil, sunflower oil.

Beverages:

Alkaline forming - alkaline water, fresh coconut water, green juices (vegetable juices), mineral water.

Acid forming - beer, black tea, coffee, soda, soft drinks, sweetened juices, wine.

Other alkalising food:

Apple cider vinegar, bee pollen, fresh fruit juice, green juices, lecithin granules, probiotic cultures, tempeh (fermented), tofu (fermented), vegetable juices, whey protein powder.

Other acid forming substances and food:

Alcohol, aspirin, cocoa, drugs (medicinal), drugs (recreational), herbicides, pesticides, some chemicals, tobacco, vinegar.

*Foods marked with an asterisk may be borderline, because on some lists they are acidic and on others, they are alkaline.

You can test yourself with litmus paper to determine your pH. A little book of 80 test strips is just pennies on eBay.

Saliva has an optimum pH of 7.5, but you should only test yourself at least 2 hours after eating.

Urine should have a pH of 7.4 mid morning, but will only be 6.5 when you first wake up, because it is more concentrated.

Insulin Potentiation

Cancer cells have many more insulin receptors than normal cells. If you eat sugar, and your pancreas releases insulin (which tells your cells to store the sugar), then the cancer cells are able to absorb much more sugar than other cells.

If you lower a person's blood sugar to 50mg/dl, or even as low as 30mg/dl, then the starving tumour is very receptive to receiving more sugar.

This also increases the cancer cells' vulnerability to low doses of chemotherapy - allowing much less to work in a much more targeted way.

After this process, the patient can be brought back up to normal blood sugar levels and then exposed to hyperthermia, which also increases the effectiveness of the chemotherapy. Chemotherapy loaded cancer cells exposed to hyperthermia for around 90 minutes are often significantly damaged, and this has been used to effectively treat brain cancers, pancreatic cancers, lung cancer, sarcoma and more, at clinics in Germany.

Metronomic Treatment

Research has shown that if a cancer cell within a tumour is positioned any more than 6 cancer cells away from a blood vessel, it dies, because the other cells steal away the nutrition for themselves. This restricts tumour thickness to just 1mm thick, unless it has a dedicated blood supply.

In the later stages of the development of a tumour, the cancer cells start to release growth factors that can trigger the growth of new blood vessels to feed the tumour. This is called angiogenisis

- the production of new additional blood vessels, from the existing blood vessels.

If you can prevent the development of blood vessels within a tumour, or decrease the blood supply, then you can inhibit tumour growth.

It has been found that this can be done by using angiogenesis inhibitors at regular intervals, hence the term meteronomic.

There are perhaps as many as 500 different known angiogenesis inhibitors. Many of these naturally occur in food. A list of natural angiogenesis inhibitors, that are contained within the superfoods listed in this book, includes:

- Aloe Vera leaf and whole extracts
- Antioxidants (vitamins A, C, E; selenium, zinc, carotenoids, flavonoids, coenzyme Q10, N-acetylcysteine, lipoic acid)
- Epigallocatechin-3 gallate (in green tea)
- Curcumin (in Turmeric / Curry)
- Garlic
- 6-Gingerol (in Ginger)
- Ginkgo biloba (ginkgolide B)
- Liquorice / Licorice
- Omega-3 fatty acids (eicosapentaenoic acid, docosahexaenoic acid)
- Resveratrol (in grape skins)
- Proanthocyanidin (in grape seeds, hazelnuts and persimmons)
- Quercetin (apples, apricots, barley, blackberries, broccoli, cherries, onions, tomatoes, watercress)
- Soy isoflavones

Rick Simpson and hemp oil

Rick Simpson is a major proponent of the curative effects of hemp oil. Whilst he is not alone in his field, he has been treating patients for several years with the essential oil of the hemp plant.

Rick claims successful treatment of several thousand patients, a number of which have provided testimonials on his website http://phoenixtears.ca

It is difficult to determine how and why he gets the results that he does, particularly for cancer patients, but given that essential oils (in general) have a very high frequency, perhaps part of its function relates to the findings of Dr Rife? An alternative theory involves the body's natural production of melatonin, and the influence of hemp oil on that mechanism.

I must point out that in many countries and jurisdictions, hemp or cannabis or marijuana, or whatever you prefer to call it, is illegal.

Legislation aside, I also draw a distinction where workplace and road safety is concerned. Evidence suggests that the use of illegal drugs, including cannabis, is inappropriate where the user is responsible for their own safety and the safety of those around them.

That aside, whilst I am not endorsing the use of hemp oil as a treatment, I am more than willing to provide an open platform for any potential cancer treatment to be discussed and considered, along with its supporting evidence.

In Rick's own words...

"Due to its harmless nature as a medicine, hemp oil is in a class all by itself. Even something like aspirin tablets that are looked upon as being harmless by the public cause thousands of deaths worldwide each year.

Hemp oil promotes full body healing and raises melatonin levels thousands of times higher than normal. When the pineal gland produces vast amounts of melatonin, it causes no harm to the body but it is very hard on the condition you are suffering from and indeed, can eliminate it. From what I can gather, all this along with your PH being raised while the oil is detoxifying your body we think causes the healing effect of this medication.

Over the years people have come to me who after years of treatment by the medical system did not even have a diagnosis for their conditions. But the oil exercised its amazing healing power and their medical problems were solved.

Another aspect of the use of hemp as medicine is its anti-aging properties. As we age, our vital organs deteriorate and of course this impairs the function of these organs. Hemp oil rejuvenates vital organs. Even in small doses. It is very common for people to report to me that they feel 20 to 30 years younger after only ingesting the oil for a short time.

What other medicine works on everything and in many cases can cure thought-to-be incurable conditions? What else can heal diabetic ulcers, skin cancers or heal third degree burns in no time, leaving no scars?

Myself and many others have gone through reams of so-called scientific studies which I found to be mostly double-talk and most of these studies were about synthetic THC which bears little resemblance to natural THC and its associated cannabinoids found in the hemp plant.

After studying all this scientific jargon, I had learned what amounted to nothing. But the oil continued to work the miracles, so who was I to question it?

I had just about given up hope that we would ever find out why the oil worked so well for all these different medical conditions. But recently a lady named Batya Stark has provided me with what I think are all the missing pieces to the puzzle.

She has sent me a great deal of information about melatonin and the pineal gland which produces it. It seems that the pineal gland is in the driver's seat when it comes to healing our bodies. The melatonin it produces is an essential part of healing. When the function of the pineal gland is impaired, it produces much less melatonin and therefore we become sick and diseased.

Studies have been released that show people suffering from cancer have low levels of melatonin in their bodies. Also studies have shown that just smoking hemp can raise the melatonin levels in our bodies. So one can only imagine what the oil, that is in a concentrated state, can do to increase melatonin levels.

As we age, we acidify, and cancer thrives in an acidic environment. So bringing the body's PH level up is very important when you are suffering from cancer and many other conditions. The oil works to do this.

Many hemp magazines are now telling their readers how to heal themselves with this wonderful medicine. If governments want to live in denial, it will be short-lived. We are gaining tens of thousands of followers every day. You cannot stop the truth.

Hemp oil has a very high success rate in the treatment of cancer. Unfortunately, many people who come to me have been badly damaged by the medical system with their chemo and radiation, etc. The damage such treatments cause have a lasting effect and people who have suffered the effects of such treatments are the hardest to cure." - Rick Simpson of http://phoenixtears.ca

You can learn more about this form of therapy, including video tutorials, interviews, lectures, testimonials and more at http://phoenixtears.ca

Or visit:

http://www.CancerUncensored.com/alternative-medicine

Further reading

The cancer treatment battlefield is littered with the fallen practitioners who have frequently been destroyed by the not so "friendly fire" of the system itself.

Whilst I fully appreciate that mainstream medicine must not be overtaken or undermined by "quacks", a better mechanism should exist to research new findings, rather than brush them off with instant dismissal, or the current demand for colossal levels of study data, when there is clearly no funding for this.

I just hope that the damage hasn't already been done, where new pioneers are too afraid to fight the system, having seen what happens to people who do.

Of course, the number of practitioners who may have had valid input to give, greatly exceeds the scope of this book. Therefore, further reading is warranted for the following doctors, researchers and healers:

Doctors Coley, Hoffer, Burzynski, Gerson, Ivy, Burton, Manner, Revici, Hamer, Issels, Beres, Moerman, Pallares, Nichols, and Willner; scientists / researchers such as Warburg, Rife, Koch, Reams, Naessens, Beljansky, Kelley, Krebs, Stone, Beard, Budwig, Cantwell, Livingstone, Beres, Lakhovsky; and healers such as Keller, Shulze, Breuss, Kushi, Binzel, Hoxsey, Caisse, Wigmore, Vonderplanitz and more.

Conclusion

Just as there is no single cause of cancer, we must perhaps acknowledge that there is no single treatment that will be universally effective.

There are many potential treatments which could be of benefit. All we need is some unbiased focus on research, rather than the apparent exclusion due to vested interests.

Ultimately, the most potent weapon against cancer is already in our hands, in the form of prevention.

We simply need to apply what science has already told us, in the form of a good diet, exercise and avoiding toxins.

Have you ever read the book, or seen the film "Alive"?

It is an extraordinary tale, based upon a true story. In 1972, 45 people travelling across the Andes, on Uruguayan Air Force Flight 571, crash landed in the mountains. Rescuers were unable to locate them, so after a number of days, they assumed the worst and called off the search.

This meant that the survivors of the crash were stranded in the snow and ice with no food for 72 days. The only hope of survival was for the living to eat the deceased passengers, many of which were friends and family. Only 16 survivors made it back alive.

It is incredible to see what people can do to survive if they have the will.

As graphic and unpleasant as the thought might be, I want you to think about it for a moment. Think what it took for them to survive.

Could you do that if it meant the difference between you seeing your family again or not?

Could you do that if it meant that you got to watch your grandchildren grow up?

Well, this is the question you should also be asking about your current lifestyle. Could you make the changes necessary to not only survive, but to age with grace?

Fortunately, throughout the course of this book I have highlighted that preventing 85% of cancer is as simple as the following:

1. Eat a wide variety of fruit, vegetables, nuts, seeds and fish. With raw, organic food options being preferable. Supplement with enzymes whenever you cannot eat raw.

2. Avoid toxic processed food options, including alcohol, processed flour, refined sugars, genetically modified foods, artificial sweeteners, preservatives and processed meats.

3. Avoid toxic environmental factors such as smoking, radon, heavy metals, radiation, chemicals, excessive sun exposure, herbicides and pesticides.

4. Actively seek out exercise, stress relieving activities, forgiveness, laughter, relationships and social ties. Spend time with those you LOVE!

If I gave these options to the 16 survivors of Flight 571, do you think they could do it to survive?

...Well so can you!

Make a start today. Even if you add one new thing each week, that is 52 changes in a year that will last you a lifetime.

But don't make these changes so you won't die... Make these changes so you can LIVE! Live to your fullest potential, and live so you can make a difference in this world.

I sincerely wish you the best of luck in your journey, and hope that like myself, you will help to spread the word.

Kindest regards as always

Chris.

Christopher C. Evans
Author of Cancer Uncensored
www.CancerUncensored.com

p.s. Please make use of the cheat sheets at the end of this book and tell your friends and loved ones about the simple changes they can make too!

"May your joys be as bright as the morning, your years of happiness as numerous as the stars in the heavens, and your troubles be but shadows that fade in the sunlight of love." - An old English blessing.

The Lazy Guide To Cancer Prevention

Food sources you should eat daily

Try to increase the number of fresh fruit and vegetables you eat - even if you only hit your "five-a-day" portion levels, you will be ahead of over 75% of Americans!

The easy way is to get yourself a good blender. This allows you to make fruit smoothies, which you can sneak vegetables into without having to taste them. Spinach, kale, and other salad greens can be consumed with ease if you add apple, banana or oranges and some fresh fruit juice. Even just 3 times per week will help, but daily is better. It is easy to fit 7 or 8 portions into a drink.

If you get yourself a good blender, (or a separate nut grinder), you can also create a mix of raw Brazil nuts, walnuts, almonds, pumpkin seeds, flaxseeds, sunflower seeds and sesame seeds. You can even add hazelnuts, pistachio nuts and dried blackberries and goji berries for more benefits. Grind them and sprinkle them on your meals. Be generous with the quantity you put on your food. I buy all my items online, so you don't have to go to the supermarket for it. Visit:

http://www.CancerUncensored.com/recommended-products

Alternatively, just eat them raw, as a snack or as a delicious cereal with coconut milk. This is great with added dried apricots.

For best health benefits, choose cruciferous or dark green leafy vegetables, such as kale, broccoli, cabbage, cauliflower, and any orange or red fruit and vegetables.

Try to include oily fish in your diet at least once per week or supplement daily with organic flaxseed oil.

If blending fruit and vegetables is too much like hard work, then use Living Fuel for a real nutrition blast. Living Fuel Inc, make a supplement called "SuperGreens" and an alternative called "SuperBerry Ultimate" formula. This is a meal replacement powder that has the highest antioxidant ratings of any food on the planet.

The formula contains all of the essential vitamins, minerals, essential fatty acids, probiotics, enzymes, antioxidants and plant compounds you should need.

On top of that, it contains all 10 essential amino acids from plant sources, (in a ratio very similar to egg), carbohydrates, fibre and healthy fats. It is the only meal replacement supplement I know of that you could live off indefinitely. Each serving contains the equivalent of 12 of your "five a day" minimum fruit and vegetable quota. So even half a serving is good for you!

Based upon my daily experience, I am not a big fan of the flavour (if only mixed with water), with the superberry version being an improvement on the supergreens version, but if mixed with fruit juice, coconut milk or blended with fruit it is barely detectable and after a while you grow to like it.

Check it out:

http://www.CancerUncensored.com/living-fuel

As a general rule, you should try to eat some foods raw, but if you do cook anything, you should steam it or cook only with cold-pressed oils such as olive oil or coconut oil.

Other nutritious foods such as mushrooms, and other items in the A to Z list of super foods should also be consumed as part of an assortment of meals spread over the week. Variety is the key to ensure that you cover all of your nutritional requirements.

Be sure to drink plenty of filtered water - at least 2 litres per day. Preferably alkaline water from a Keosan water filter.

Supplementation:

Either consume a serving of Living Fuel, or else use...

- A good solid multivitamin and mineral tablet.
- 1000 mg timed release vitamin C tablet.
- 1000 mg organic flaxseed oil.
- A calcium, magnesium and zinc supplement.
- Lactobacillus acidophilus (at least 2 billion viable organisms per capsule).
- Digestive enzyme capsules with your cooked meals (the best formulas have up to a dozen different enzymes).
- A SuperGreens tablet - containing wheatgrass, Spiro Lena, chlorella and other antioxidant rich plants.

Food sources you should eat less of, or avoid.

Avoid:

- Genetically Modified Foods (GMOs), including maize (corn), wheat, barley, kidney beans, soya beans, sugar beet,etc.
- Foods high in processed sugar - foods with a high glycaemic index not only cause premature ageing of your tissues, but they also strip the minerals from your bones and teeth.
- Preservatives / irradiation - eat fresh, preferably raw, and avoid foods preserved with nitrates or phosphates.
- Artificial colours, flavours and preservatives, including additives such as monosodium glutamate.
- Artificial sweeteners, such as aspartame, acesulfame K (or acesulfame potassium), and saccharin.
- Trans fats or hydrogenated fats or any other oils that have not been cold-pressed.

- Acrylamides in fast foods and bakery products.
- Wheat - or any other food which may cause a food intolerance for allergy response (this suppresses your body's ability to fight cancer).
- Cured meats.
- Red meats.
- Mass produced cows' milk - opt for coconut milk or almond milk instead - worst case scenario, organic milk.
- Cut down on Coffee.

Habits and environmental factors you should seek more of.

- Exercise - at a minimum find a reason to move around for 10 minutes every few hours. Go to the toilet, fetch a drink, go upstairs. Anything. The movement moves your lymphatic system, which boosts your immune system and helps you eliminate toxins. It also stimulates antioxidant production. Preferably, do this every hour. Hard exercise improves your heart health, but movement purges your lymphatic system because it doesn't have a pump.
- Moderate sun exposure - the boosting of vitamin D helps to stimulate your immune system.
- Increase your intake of oxygen - several times a day, deliberately take at least 10 very deep breaths (in and out) to hyper-oxygenate your system. Cancer cells respond very poorly to elevated levels of oxygen.
- Get plenty of sleep - getting 8 hours a day of sleep ensures you reduce your stress levels, and it is during sleep that your body enters its most intense period of growth and repair, building new proteins, replacing damaged cells and boosting your immune system.

Habits and environmental factors you should seek to avoid.

- Smoking.
- Cut down on alcohol.
- Limit the time you spend wearing a bra.
- Illegal drugs.
- Genetically Modified Foods - so bad they were worth mentioning twice!
- Radon gas - you can check your home using simple test kits.
- Diesel or petrol exhaust fumes - always wear gloves when you are fuelling your vehicle and try not to breathe in any of the fumes (although this is easier said than done).
- Food intolerances or allergens.
- Dental toxicities - from undiagnosed infections, root canals, mercury-based fillings or nickel crowns.
- Heavy metals - filter your water, and conduct a heavy metal detox each year.
- Pesticides or herbicides - try to buy organic produce, or wash your vegetables and fruit thoroughly before consuming them.
- Environmental carcinogens such as dioxins.
- Parasites - conduct a parasite cleanse once or twice per year.

Using your psychology to give you the edge.

- Positive thinking reaps rewards. Try self-help books, hypnosis, self hypnosis CDs, guided meditation, affirmations, subliminal CDs and anything you can to reinforce a positive outlook.
- Laughter - laughter not only increases your happiness, but it also triggers a boost to your immune system, a decrease in stress hormone levels and an increase in endorphins (which are the body's natural feel-good chemicals).

- Become super social - longevity studies show that being sociable significantly increases lifespan.
- Find ways to eliminate emotional stresses, such as meditation, yoga, massage, walks in nature, music and socialising.
- Address any suppressed or unresolved anger issues or emotional issues. Do not bottle anything up inside you - even if it means writing a one-way letter to everyone who ever upset you. You don't need to send it, just write it, so you can 'let go'.

The Dedicated Guide To Cancer Prevention

Food sources you should eat daily

Try to increase the number of fresh fruit and vegetables you eat - even if you only hit your "five-a-day" portion levels, you will be ahead of over 75% of Americans!

You should aim to hit your five-a-day purely within your main meals, then add to that with smoothies and juices, to painlessly bump your score up to 8 to 10 per day.

For this, you will need a good blender. This allows you to make delicious fruit smoothies, which you can sneak vegetables into without having to taste them. Tomatoes, spinach, kale, and other salad greens can be consumed with ease on a daily basis if you add apple, banana, berries or oranges and some fresh fruit juice. Even just 3 times per week will help, but daily is better. You would be surprised how easy it is to fit 7 or 8 portions into a drink.

If you get yourself a good blender, (or a separate nut grinder), you can also create a mix of raw Brazil nuts, walnuts, almonds, pumpkin seeds, flaxseeds, sunflower seeds and sesame seeds. You can even add hazelnuts, pistachio nuts and dried blackberries and goji berries for more benefits. Buy raw and organic.

Grind them and sprinkle them on your meals. Be generous with the quantity you put on your food. I also do the same with organic flaxseed. Brown linseed or flaxseed, (same thing), has slightly more omega-3 oil than golden flaxseed, but I use them both.

I buy all my items online, so you don't have to go to the supermarket for it. Visit:

http://www.CancerUncensored.com/recommended-products

Alternatively, just eat them raw, as a snack or as a delicious cereal with coconut milk. This is great with added dried apricots, and the almonds will suppress your hunger.

For best health benefits, choose cruciferous or dark green leafy vegetables, such as kale, broccoli, cabbage, cauliflower, several times per week and try to consume any and all orange or red fruit and vegetables. Try to mix it up, so you get some great variety over the course of the week.

Try to include oily fish in your diet at least once per week, preferably twice, and supplement daily with organic flaxseed oil, 1000mg minimum.

If blending fruit and vegetables is too much like hard work, then use Living Fuel for a real nutrition blast. I always add it to my smoothies to ensure balanced nutrition and easy digestion. Living Fuel Inc, make a supplement called "SuperGreens" and an alternative called "SuperBerry Ultimate" formula. This is a meal replacement powder that has the highest antioxidant ratings of any food on the planet.

The formula contains all of the essential vitamins, minerals, essential fatty acids, probiotics, enzymes, antioxidants and plant compounds you should need.

On top of that, it contains all 10 essential amino acids from plant sources, (in a ratio very similar to egg), carbohydrates, fibre and healthy fats. It is the only meal replacement supplement I know of that you could live off indefinitely. Each serving contains the equivalent of 12 of your "five a day" minimum fruit and vegetable quota. So even half a serving is good for you!

Based upon my daily experience, I am not a big fan of the flavour (if only mixed with water), with the superberry version being an improvement on the supergreens version, but if mixed with fruit juice, coconut milk or blended with fruit it is barely detectable and after a while you grow to like it.

Check it out:

http://www.CancerUncensored.com/living-fuel

As a general rule, you should try to eat as many foods as you can in their raw state, to preserve the nutrition and enzymes, but if you do cook anything, steam it or cook only with cold-pressed oils such as olive oil or coconut oil.

Other nutritious foods such as mushrooms, and other items in the A to Z list of super foods should also be consumed as part of an assortment of meals spread over the week. Variety is the key to ensure that you cover all of your nutritional requirements.

Be sure to drink plenty of filtered water - at least 2 litres per day. Preferably alkaline water from a Keosan water filter or something similar.

Supplementation:

Either consume a serving of Living Fuel, or else use...

- A good solid multivitamin and mineral tablet.
- 1000 mg timed release vitamin C tablet.
- 1000 mg organic flaxseed oil.
- A calcium, magnesium and zinc supplement.
- Lactobacillus acidophilus (at least 2 billion viable organisms per capsule).
- Digestive enzyme capsules with your cooked meals (the best formulas have up to a dozen different enzymes).
- A SuperGreens tablet - containing wheatgrass, Spiro Lena, chlorella and other antioxidant rich plants.

For the ultimate in prevention, you can add various other supplements, including capsules of substances shown to kill cancer cells, or shrink tumours in lab, animal and human studies. The following natural compounds have no harmful side effects - gingerols from ginger, curcumin from turmeric, capsaicin from peppers, proanthocyanidins in grape seed extract, EGCG from green tea, allicin from garlic, and ellagic acid from pomegranate seed extract.

Food sources you should eat less of, or avoid.

Avoid:

- Genetically Modified Foods (GMOs), including maize (corn), wheat, barley, kidney beans, soya beans, sugar beet,etc.
- Foods high in processed sugar - foods with a high glycaemic index not only cause premature ageing of your tissues, but they also strip the minerals from your bones and teeth.
- Preservatives / irradiation - eat fresh, preferably raw, and avoid foods preserved with nitrates or phosphates.
- Artificial colours, flavours and preservatives, including additives such as monosodium glutamate.
- Artificial sweeteners, such as aspartame, acesulfame K (or acesulfame potassium), and saccharin.
- Trans fats or hydrogenated fats or any other oils that have not been cold-pressed.
- Acrylamides in fast foods and bakery products.
- Wheat - or any other food which may cause a food intolerance for allergy response (this suppresses your body's ability to fight cancer).
- Farmed fish - ocean caught fish such as Alaskan salmon is fantastic, but farmed fish may contain heavy metals.
- Cured meats.
- Red meats.
- Economy chicken, which may well have been fed GMO corn. Opt for organic chicken or turkey, or better yet eat fish and organic eggs as your only animal protein.

- Mass produced cows' milk - opt for coconut milk or almond milk instead - worst case scenario, organic milk.
- Coffee.
- Any foods you may have an intolerance to. Carry out a food intolerance test to find out which ones cause a problem for you.
- If you currently have cancer, or have a family history, there is an argument for going vegetarian, or pescetarian (where you still eat fish). In a perfect world, vegan, but this takes planning and dedication to do it healthily. I advise you to skip to the Survivor's guide if you have been diagnosed.

Habits and environmental factors you should seek more of.

- Exercise - 30 minutes at least 3 times per week. Feel free to vary the intensity and activity, but the exercise moves your lymphatic system, which boosts your immune system and helps you eliminate toxins. It also stimulates antioxidant production. Preferably, find a reason to move around for 10 minutes every hour.
- Moderate sun exposure - the boosting of vitamin D helps to stimulate your immune system.
- Drink plenty of water, preferably well filtered alkaline water. Bottled water is better than tap water, but unfortunately it still may well contain plasticisers / bisphenol A from the material the bottle is made from. Get yourself a serious water filter, which also means that you can cook and make hot drinks with filtered water.
- Dry skin brushing - this helps to remove uric acid crystals from your skin and eases the burden on your kidneys and liver.
- Massage - not only does this help to move the fluid in your lymphatic system, but the relaxation and well-being reduces your levels of stress (which causes additional free radicals). You may also wish to consider colonic massage

(where the abdomen is massaged externally to stimulate the shedding of built-up faecal matter. You can lose a dress size in a single session!).
- Increase your intake of oxygen - several times a day, deliberately take at least 10 very deep breaths (in and out) to hyper-oxygenate your system. Cancer cells respond very poorly to elevated levels of oxygen. You can also purchase an oxygen bar, in order to give yourself deliberate boosts of oxygen.
- Get plenty of sleep - getting 8 hours a day of sleep ensures you reduce your stress levels, and it is during sleep that your body enters its most intense period of growth and repair, building new proteins, replacing damaged cells and boosting your immune system.

Habits and environmental factors you should seek to avoid.

- Smoking.
- Limit alcohol to special occasions.
- Limit the time you spend wearing a bra.
- Illegal drugs.
- Genetically Modified Foods - so bad they were worth mentioning twice!
- Radon gas - you can check your home using simple test kits.
- Diesel or petrol exhaust fumes - always wear gloves when you are fuelling your vehicle and try not to breathe in any of the fumes (although this is easier said than done).
- Food intolerances or allergens.
- Dental toxicities - from undiagnosed infections, root canals, mercury-based fillings or nickel crowns.
- Heavy metals - filter your water, and conduct a heavy metal detox each year.

- Pesticides or herbicides - try to buy organic produce, or wash your vegetables and fruit thoroughly before consuming them.
- Environmental carcinogens such as dioxins.
- Parasites - conduct a parasite cleanse once or twice per year.

Using your psychology to give you the edge.

- Positive thinking reaps rewards. Try self-help books, hypnosis, self hypnosis CDs, guided meditation, affirmations, subliminal CDs and anything you can to reinforce a positive outlook.
- Laughter - laughter not only increases your happiness, but it also triggers a boost to your immune system, a decrease in stress hormone levels and an increase in endorphins (which are the body's natural feel-good chemicals).
- Become super social - longevity studies show that being sociable significantly increases lifespan.
- Find ways to eliminate emotional stresses, such as meditation, yoga, massage, walks in nature, music and socialising.
- Address any suppressed or unresolved anger issues or emotional issues. Do not bottle anything up inside you - even if it means writing a one-way letter to everyone who ever upset you. You don't need to send it, just write it, so you can 'let go'.

The Survivors Guide To Cancer Prevention and Survival

Food sources you should eat daily

Create a mix of raw Brazil nuts, walnuts, almonds, pumpkin seeds, flaxseeds, sunflower seeds and sesame seeds. You can even add hazelnuts, pistachio nuts and dried blackberries and goji berries for more benefits. Grind them with a nut grinder and sprinkle them on every single meal you eat. Be generous with the quantity you put on your food. I also do the same with organic flaxseed. Brown linseed or flaxseed, (same thing), has slightly more omega-3 oil than golden flaxseed, but I use them both.

Alternatively, just eat your favourite nuts raw, with every meal. I have found that you can grind them with a nut grinder, then pour on coconut milk or almond milk to make a delicious cereal. This is great with added dried apricots.

Every single day, in addition to the nuts and seeds listed above, you should consume some quantity of each of the following:

Organic cold processed Whey protein, broccoli, kale, spinach, tomatoes, oily fish, sweet potato, cold-pressed extra virgin olive oil or olives, apples, blackberries or blueberries - all red fruits, vegetables and berries are great. If you're having trouble consuming enough of these foods, invest in a good-quality food processor and blend combinations of them into a smoothie for quick consumption. Blendtec, Turbochef or Vitamix blenders can turn almost anything to liquid, so be creative. Beetroot juice is also very helpful for its detoxifying and oxygen boosting properties. The fruit will help disguise anything you don't like.

I also blend in flaxseeds, aloe vera juice, organic bee pollen, and Living Fuel for a real nutrition blast.

Visit the following page for a list of products I use:

http://www.CancerUncensored.com/recommended-products

This kind of diet is not cheap, particularly if you are purchasing organic products, but you cannot put a price on your health or your survival.

As a general rule, you should eat raw, but if you do cook anything, you should steam it, and only cook with cold-pressed oils such as olive oil or coconut oil.

Other nutritious foods such as mushrooms, and other items in the A to Z list of super foods should also be consumed as part of an assortment of meals spread over the week. Variety is the key to ensure that you cover all of your nutritional requirements.

Be sure to drink plenty of water - at least 2 litres per day. Preferably alkaline water from a Keosan water filter or something similar.

Supplementation:

- A good solid multivitamin and mineral tablet, or Living Fuel.
- 1000 mg timed release vitamin C tablet twice per day.
- 1000 mg organic flaxseed oil twice per day.
- A calcium, magnesium and zinc supplement.
- Lactobacillus acidophilus (at least 2 billion viable organisms per capsule).
- Digestive enzyme capsules with each main meal - especially if cooked, (the best formulas have up to a dozen different enzymes).
- SuperGreens formula - containing wheatgrass, Spiro Lena, chlorella and other antioxidant rich plants.

- (Controversial) Apricot kernels containing vitamin B17.

All of the supplementation items above (except the vitamin B17) can be replaced with a single supplement called "SuperGreens" by a company called Living Fuel Inc. They also offer a "SuperBerry Ultimate" formula. These formulations have the highest antioxidant ratings of any food on the planet. The formula contains all of the essential vitamins, minerals, essential fatty acids, probiotics, enzymes, antioxidants and plant compounds you should need.

On top of that, it contains all 10 essential amino acids from plant sources, (in a ratio very similar to egg), carbohydrates, fibre and healthy fats. It is the only meal replacement supplement I know of that you could live off indefinitely. Each serving contains the equivalent of 12 of your "five a day" minimum fruit and vegetable quota.

Based upon my daily experience, I am not a big fan of the flavour (if only mixed with water), with the superberry version being an improvement on the supergreens version, but if mixed with fruit juice, or blended with fruit it is barely detectable and after a while you grow to like it.

I blend it with fresh juice, fruit and my organic cocoa flavoured whey protein to give it a chocolate orange flavour whilst retaining the natural ingredients. Alternatively, I mix it with coconut milk and the same cocoa enhanced whey protein to give it a chocolate milkshake effect. But let's be honest, this product is so good for you, I would drink it however it tasted! Better to use blended fruit and water with it, rather than store-bought juice, because the fibre slows down the absorption of the fruit sugar, and they have not been pasteurised.

If you load it with berries and other fruit, you can add in spinach, kale and a range of other greens without impacting upon the flavour. It is the easiest way I know to get so many vegetables into people who don't normally like them! Great for kids.

Check it out:

http://www.CancerUncensored.com/living-fuel

For the ultimate in prevention, you can add various other supplements, including capsules of substances shown to kill cancer cells, or shrink tumours in lab, animal and human studies. The following natural compounds have no harmful side effects - gingerols from ginger, curcumin from turmeric, capsaicin from peppers, proanthocyanidins in grape seed extract, EGCG from green tea, allicin from garlic, and ellagic acid from pomegranate seed extract.

If you have been diagnosed with cancer, please see the Alternative Therapy Checklist at the end of this guide for dosage information.

Food sources you should eat less of, or avoid.

Avoid:

- Genetically Modified Foods (GMOs), including maize (corn), wheat, barley, kidney beans, soya beans, sugar beet,etc.
- Foods high in processed sugar - foods with a high glycaemic index not only cause premature ageing of your tissues, but they also strip the minerals from your bones and teeth.
- Preservatives / irradiation - eat fresh, preferably raw, and avoid foods preserved with nitrates or phosphates.
- Artificial colours, flavours and preservatives, including additives such as monosodium glutamate.
- Artificial sweeteners, such as aspartame, acesulfame K (or acesulfame potassium), and saccharin.
- Trans fats or hydrogenated fats or any other oils that have not been cold-pressed.
- Acrylamides in fast foods and bakery products.

- Wheat - or any other food which may cause a food intolerance for allergy response (this suppresses your body's ability to fight cancer).
- Farmed fish - ocean caught fish such as Alaskan salmon is fantastic, but farmed fish may contain heavy metals.
- Cured meats.
- Red meats.
- Economy chicken, which may well have been fed GMO corn. Opt for organic chicken or turkey, or better yet eat fish and organic eggs as your only animal protein.
- Mass produced cows' milk - opt for coconut milk or almond milk instead - worst case scenario, organic milk.
- Coffee.
- Any foods you may have an intolerance to. Carry out a food intolerance test to find out which ones cause a problem for you.
- If you have breast cancer or prostate cancer, it may be advisable to avoid soy-based products because they influence your hormone levels.
- If you currently have cancer, there is an argument for going vegan. This takes planning and dedication to do it healthily.

Habits and environmental factors you should seek more of.

- Exercise - 45 min per day. Feel free to vary the intensity and activity, but the exercise moves your lymphatic system, which boosts your immune system and helps you eliminate toxins. It also stimulates antioxidant production. Preferably, find a reason to move around for 10 minutes every hour.
- Moderate sun exposure - the boosting of vitamin D helps to stimulate your immune system.
- Drink plenty of water, preferably well filtered alkaline water. Bottled water is better than tap water, but

unfortunately it still may well contain plasticisers / bisphenol A from the material the bottle is made from. Get yourself a serious water filter, which also means that you can cook and make hot drinks with filtered water.
- Dry skin brushing - this helps to remove uric acid crystals from your skin and eases the burden on your kidneys and liver.
- Massage - not only does this help to move the fluid in your lymphatic system, but the relaxation and well-being reduces your levels of stress (which causes additional free radicals). You may also wish to consider colonic massage (where the abdomen is massaged externally to stimulate the shedding of built-up faecal matter. You can lose a dress size in a single session!).
- Infrared sauna - stimulates the mitochondria in your cells to release energy more efficiently and also helps your body to detoxify, thereby reducing the stress on your liver and kidneys. It increases heart rate and can act like exercise on the body, even though you just sit there.
- Increase your intake of oxygen - several times a day, deliberately take at least 10 very deep breaths (in and out) to hyper-oxygenate your system. Cancer cells respond very poorly to elevated levels of oxygen. You can also purchase an oxygen bar, in order to give yourself deliberate boosts of oxygen.
- Get plenty of sleep - getting 8 hours a day of sleep ensures you reduce your stress levels, and it is during sleep that your body enters its most intense period of growth and repair, building new proteins, replacing damaged cells and boosting your immune system.

Habits and environmental factors you should seek to avoid.

- Smoking.
- Alcohol.
- Limit the time you spend wearing a bra.

- Illegal drugs.
- Genetically Modified Foods - so bad they were worth mentioning twice!
- Radon gas - you can check your home using simple test kits.
- Diesel or petrol exhaust fumes - always wear gloves when you are fuelling your vehicle and try not to breathe in any of the fumes (although this is easier said than done).
- Food intolerances or allergens.
- Dental toxicities - from undiagnosed infections, root canals, mercury-based fillings or nickel crowns.
- Heavy metals - filter your water, and conduct a heavy metal detox each year.
- Pesticides or herbicides - try to buy organic produce, or wash your vegetables and fruit thoroughly before consuming them.
- Environmental carcinogens such as dioxins.
- Parasites - conduct a parasite cleanse once or twice per year.

Using your psychology to give you the edge.

- Positive thinking reaps rewards. Try self-help books, hypnosis, self hypnosis CDs, guided meditation, affirmations, subliminal CDs and anything you can to reinforce a positive outlook.
- Laughter - laughter not only increases your happiness, but it also triggers a boost to your immune system, a decrease in stress hormone levels and an increase in endorphins (which are the body's natural feel-good chemicals).
- Build a support structure around you with family members and friends.
- Become super social - longevity studies show that being sociable significantly increases lifespan.

- Find ways to eliminate emotional stresses, such as meditation, yoga, massage, walks in nature, music and socialising.
- Do not underestimate the placebo effect - countless studies have shown that belief alters your reality. If you BELIEVE you will get well or stay well, you have a statistically greater chance. Work on your mindset, and use visualisation to make it a reality.
- Address any suppressed or unresolved anger issues or emotional issues. Do not bottle anything up inside you - even if it means writing a one-way letter to everyone who ever upset you. You don't need to send it, just write it, so you can 'let go'.

Alternative Therapy Checklist

The following treatments and procedures may not be mainstream medicine, but they are based on research and solid science. Many do not conflict with conventional treatment, so you should certainly investigate all of your options. I have personally seen individuals who had been written-off as incurable/terminal who have had a complete recovery using science-based alternative medicine.

- Oxygen / Ozone Autohaemotherapy - cancer cells respond very poorly to high levels of oxygen.
- Whole-body or partial hyperthermia - tumours are more susceptible to damage from increased heat than healthy tissue.
- Megadose vitamin C intravenous infusions - cancer cells are negatively impacted by high levels of vitamins C.
- High levels of fish oil or flaxseed oil - correcting our imbalance of omega-3 and omega-6 has a suppression effect on tumours. See the Budwig diet in the Alternative Medicine section of Cancer Uncensored.
- Vitamin B17 - this compound is harmless for healthy tissue, but cancer cells break it down, releasing a

molecule of cyanide directly within the cancer cell, making it a highly targeted therapy.
- Eliminating the causes of persistent allergies and food intolerances. If your allergic responses are fired up continuously, it depletes your body's ability to respond to disease and cancer.
- Eliminating parasites - a parasitic load can trigger all manner of allergic and inflammatory responses.
- Have dental toxicities removed - mercury fillings, nickel crowns, root canals, etc.
- General detox and cleansing, in the order of colon cleansing, parasite cleansing, kidney cleansing, liver and gall bladder cleanse, heavy metal detox, followed by blood cleanse. This process gets your body back to an initial baseline of health, breaking the negative cycle that has built up due to toxins, heavy metals and a general overload of your system.
- Assorted biochemical tests - this determines your baseline levels of health, and also helps the practitioner to monitor the effectiveness of any treatments that you undertake. It can also highlight any underlying conditions that may be contributing to, (or the cause of), your illness.
- Adhering to a predominantly vegetarian raw diet - get a good quality blender / juicer so that you can consume an additional 10-15 assorted portions of fruit / vegetables / seeds and nuts per day.
- Supplementing with substances shown to kill cancer cells, or shrink tumours in cell, animal and human studies, but which have no harmful side effects - such as capsules containing gingerols from ginger, curcumin from Turmeric, capsaicin from Peppers, proanthocyanidins in grape seed extract, EGCG from Green Tea, allicin from Garlic, and Ellagic acid from Pomegranate seed extract. Take the recommended dose on the packaging for prevention purposes.

The doses required for each of the above, in order to mirror the levels used in the various studies referenced in the A to Z of Superfoods section of this book, are as follows:

(This is not a recommendation, it is merely clarifying what the studies found effective, with no data on cross reaction or cumulative effect if used together).

- 100mg gingerols daily (same as 20g ginger root, or 500mg of 20% gingerol ginger extract).
- 400mg capsaicin 3 x per week (same as 8 habanero peppers 3 x per week).
- 500mg 95% Curcumin x 2 daily (approximately same as 30g turmeric powder).
- 100mg 95% Oligomeric Proanthocyanidins (OPCs) (from grape seed extract x 1 capsule daily).
- 400mg Green tea x 2 daily (contains total of 400mg EGCG and 8mg caffeine)
- 270mg Allicin (from garlic, found in Alliforce x 1 capsule daily)
- 200mg Ellagic acid (from 250mg pomegranate seed extract capsule containing 40% ellagic acid taken x 2 daily).

Of course, this checklist section is not exhaustive, but all of the above are based upon scientific study and could help your body to respond better to whatever form of treatment you opt for. But always check with your Doctor - especially if you are taking any medication or are about to undergo treatment.

Your Doctor is highly unlikely to recommend any of the above, so your question should perhaps be, "would it do any harm if I were to add this to my diet or treatment regime?"

To keep up-to-date with the latest news and developments, visit:

http://www.CancerUncensored.com

Copyright © 2012 . Christopher C. Evans
All rights reserved.

This book contains material protected under International and Federal Copyright laws and Treaties. Any unauthorised reprint or use of this material is prohibited.

Unauthorised duplication or distribution of this material in any form is strictly prohibited. Violators will be prosecuted to the fullest extent of the law. No part of this publication may be reproduced, stored in a retrieval system or transmitted in any form or by any means, electronic, mechanical, photocopying, recording or otherwise, without prior written permission from the author/publisher.

The author, publisher, and distributor of this product assume no responsibility for the use or misuse of this product, or for any physical or mental injury, damage and/or financial loss sustained to persons or property as a result of using this system. The liability, negligence, use, misuse or abuse of the operation of any methods, strategies, instructions or ideas contained in the material herein is the sole responsibility of the reader.

The material contained in this publication is provided for information purposes only. It does not diagnose nor treat any condition, nor replace sound medical advice from your doctor. (However, I would recommend that you always get a second opinion!).